Finding a Sacred Oasis in Grief

A resource manual for pastoral care givers

T0143294

Steven L. Jeffers PhD

and

Harold Ivan Smith DMin FT

The Institute for Spirituality in Health
Shawnee Mission Medical Center
Shawnee Mission, Kansas

CRC Press
Taylor & Francis Group
Boca Raton London New York

CRC Press is an imprint of the
Taylor & Francis Group, an **informa** business

First published 2007 by Radcliffe Publishing

Published 2016 by CRC Press
Taylor & Francis Group
6000 Broken Sound Parkway NW, Suite 300
Boca Raton, FL 33487-2742

ISBN-13: 978-1-84619-181-7 (pbk)

Visit the Taylor & Francis Web site at
http://www.taylorandfrancis.com

and the CRC Press Web site at
http://www.crcpress.com

British Library Cataloguing in Publication Data

A catalogue record for this book is available from the British Library.

Typeset by Advance Typesetting Ltd, Oxford

Contents

Foreword

John D. Morgan, PhD

It is trite to say that we live in a death/grief-denying culture, but it is nevertheless true. No one wants to admit that life and all of our relationships are limited. We accept the abstraction of our own death. But we do not have an affective consciousness of death. We do not seem to take seriously that death as the end of our possibilities, the collapse of our space and time (Flynn, 1987). As death is removed from daily consciousness, it appears to be *less appropriate* (Corr, 1979), creating more complicated grief (Rando, 1993, p. 47).

The very appearance of death has changed. We now do not admit that a death has occurred until we have a technological "proof," moving death "from the moral order to the technological order" (Cassell, 1978, p. 121). As medicine specialized, the place of death changed. Medicine was no longer practiced in the patient's home or in the doctor's office, but more and more in hospitals. The consequence of this is that dying is today seen by fewer people than it was previously. There are few role models for the realities of dying and mourning.

There are many reasons for this stance taken by our culture. As Feifel (1990) has pointed out, death denial is rooted first of all in the mind–body split taught by Descartes in the seventeenth century. This split gave energy to the scientific revolution, since bodies were studied, and conquered. At the same time, a new economic shift occurred. Capitalism taught that productivity was an end in itself, a sign of one's fundamental value. We have all benefited from the achievements of capitalism and the scientific revolution: clean water, longer and healthier life. There has been a cost, however. That cost was that the non-material matters of emotion and spirit were considered "soft," not worthy of study. These were matters better left to poets and the Church.

As long as communities worked—that is, as long as people cooperated, cared for and respected each other—the emphasis on return of capital, scientific knowledge and material things was mitigated. Social support was a daily part of life and readily found in times of crisis. In addition, faith communities provided a basic sense of the meaningfulness of individual lives.

With the lessening of the tight bonds of community and faith, people began to feel more fully the intrinsic alienation that seems to be part of materialism and capitalism. The twentieth century saw massive destruction of lives, more deaths than the rest of human history combined (Corr, 1979).

Ours does not seem to be an integrated death attitude system which would enable individuals "to think, feel and behave with respect to death in ways that they might consider to be effective and appropriate" (Kastenbaum and Aisenberg, 1972, p. 193). It does not contribute to psychological growth and alleviate fears of death and bereavement giving the sense that death is a part of a full life. Parsons indicated that an ideal death would be a coincidence of the meaning of the words—"His work is done"—for both the dying patient and the physician. The patient is "ready to go," whereas the physician has not only done the best to "save" the patient's life, but has complemented these efforts by facilitating a dignified and meaningful death (Parsons *et al.*, 1973, p. 39).

This present volume by Steven Jeffers and Harold Ivan Smith does not change our culture. What it does do is give care givers the tools to help dying and grieving persons face the best and worst that life has to offer. It is the worst, because death means the end of the attachments that make life worthwhile. It is the best, because it shows us what is truly meaningful and important in life. Mortality is a great gift if we have the knowledge and the courtesy to face it.

Jeffers and Smith are to be thanked for providing us this book and the lessons that the great traditions provide in facing mortality.

John D. Morgan, PhD
Professor Emeritus of Philosophy
Coordinator for Kings College Center for Education
about Death and Bereavement
Ontario, Canada
February 2007

About the Authors

Steven L. Jeffers, PhD, is founder and director of the Institute for Spirituality in Health at Shawnee Mission Medical Center, a regional medical center in the suburbs of Kansas City. Jeffers received a BA from Palm Beach Atlantic College, an MDiv from Midwestern Baptist Theological Seminary and a PhD from Florida State University.

Jeffers works with healthcare providers, civic, business and religious leaders of various faith traditions to advocate for the compassionate care of patients and families and the integration of spirituality into the practice of medicine. He makes presentations throughout the United States on end-of-life issues and grief ministry, among other subjects. He is an author of several books and articles.

Harold Ivan Smith is a faculty member of the American Academy of Grief. He is also a board member of the Association for Death Education and Counseling. Smith holds degrees from Scarritt College (MA) and Asbury Theological Seminary (DMin). He frequently leads workshops for hospice training events and pastoral leadership conferences nationally and internationally.

He has been the keynote speaker of the National Hospice Organization's Conference on Pastoral Care, the National Perinatal Bereavement Conference and the King's Conference on Bereavement in Canada. He was a presenter at the Third World Gathering on Bereavement, the International Conference on Care and Kindness, and the National Funeral Directors Association. Smith has published over 20 books and numerous articles on bereavement.

Acknowledgments

We are deeply indebted to and greatly appreciative of the numerous people who made substantial contributions, thus improving the quality and relevance of this book.

We want to thank those who provided information for the section on grief from some of the world's religious traditions:

- Barb McAtee—Baha'i
- Bruce Nelson—Buddhism
- Chuck Stanford—Buddhism
- Anand Bhattacharyya—Hinduism
- A. Rauf Mir, MD—Islam
- Nina Shik, RN—Judaism
- Rabbi Joshua D. Kreindler—Judaism
- Kara Hawkins—Native American.

Furthermore, Mercedes Bern-Klug's extensive work concerning final arrangements was important material for incorporation into such a work. We sincerely appreciate her consenting to allow us to reproduce some of the results from her research into this book.

Moreover, we are truly appreciative of the labor of love of several people who carefully read the manuscript and offered helpful suggestions, many of which were included in the final product: Lou Gehring, Jerry Rexin, Martha Rexin, Ivan Bartolome, Quentin Jones, Eileen Connell and John Landsberg.

In addition, we are very thankful for the serious attention that three specialists in grief and loss gave in reading the manuscript and making suggestions for improving its quality—Joy Johnson of the Centering Corporation in Omaha, Nebraska, Dr. Kenneth Doka, professor of gerontology at the Graduate School of the College of New Rochelle and Senior Consultant to the Hospice Foundation of America, and Nancy Crump, certified grief counselor of D.W. Newcomer's Sons in Kansas City, Missouri. All of these individuals are authors and speakers on the subject of bereavement. In the manuscript, the reader will find many references attributed to them as well as the incorporation of many of their suggestions for quality improvement of this work.

Finally, we are grateful to Samuel H. Turner, Sr., President and CEO of Shawnee Mission Medical Center, along with Joyce Portela, Robin Harrold, Jack Wagner, Sheri Hawkins and Peter Bath, senior administrators of Shawnee Mission Medical Center, for their encouragement and support through the many months of research for and writing of the manuscript.

Steven L. Jeffers
Harold Ivan Smith
February 2007

Introduction

Grief is something that all people have experienced multiple times in their lives. Infants grieve at the loss of a breast or bottle of milk. Children grieve when they are unable to find that favorite toy. Teenagers grieve at the breakup of young love. Similarly, married couples of various ages grieve at the dissolution of wedded union. People grieve when terminated from employment. Individuals grieve when relocating from one geographical proximity to another. Persons grieve at the loss of health. Loved ones grieve at the death of a family member or a special friend.

Grief is not confined exclusively to a situation involving one's demise. Furthermore, expressions of grief are not abnormal responses to these and other similar events. On the contrary, grief is a natural, normal, healthy process, which enables traumatized people to move through times of extreme difficulty with minimal unhealthy and lingering effects.

According to grief specialist Therese Rando (1984, p. 5), there are three general patterns of grief:

1 grief-accepting
2 grief-defying
3 grief-denying.

> *"The greatest deterrent to helping grieving people is the fact that many professionals have never dealt with their own losses or have never had a person close to them die. Thus, it becomes too painful to reach out to others, and they simply hide behind 'professionalism.''*
>
> *Nancy Crump**

The purpose of this resource manual is to provide pastoral care givers of various faith and spirituality traditions with the resources for decisive leadership in ministry with grieving persons: before a loved one's death, at the time of death, during the post-death rituals, and in the times of transition that lead to reconciliation with the death.

> *"Probably there is no greater need for a pastor's (or any pastoral care provider's) ministry in a person's life than when that person experiences the death of a loved one. No other opportunity in life gives the pastor (or any pastoral care provider) a better chance to minister to people.''*
>
> *Robert Anderson (1985, p. 254)*

Anderson's words as used here are not cliché, or intended to minimize the hurt and loss people feel at the breakup of relationships, being laid off from work, leaving behind friends/family/coworkers that results from a lengthy move (in terms of miles) to another home, or a plethora of other events which cause human suffering and pain. Rather, they do bring into clear focus the heightened degree of intensity of grief that people experience surrounding physical death.

---

*Nancy Crump is a Certified Grief Counselor and Coordinator of Aftercare Services for DW Newcomer's Sons, Kansas City, Missouri. Material from Ms Crump received through personal interview.

This book will primarily address the issue of pastoral care to dying persons, as well as those grieving the loss of a loved one through death. Morrie Schwartz's words in *Tuesdays with Morrie* articulate what we hope to accomplish in this work.

> *"I'm on the last great journey here ... and people want me to tell them what to pack."*
>
> *Morrie Schwartz (Albom, 1997, p. 33)*

A significantly large number of people in the United States alone could benefit from Professor Schwartz's words and those of pastoral care givers. According to the U. S. Census Bureau (2006), 2,443,387 people died in this country in 2002 (the last year numbers were available). If we were to arbitrarily assign the number of persons influenced by each of those deaths as only five (a substantially low estimate to say the least), that computation translates into about 12 million individuals who are directly impacted by death in the span of one year. Having said that, each one of those deaths creates, at least theoretically, an opportunity for unquestioned leadership in pastoral care responses at several junctures:

- before the death
- at the time of death
- in the interim between the death and rituals
- during the time of rituals
- in post-ritual bereavement.

> *"Reverend Thomas Nelson faced a decision one cold day. No one had come to the funeral home to pay respects; no one had come to the cemetery. Nelson conferred with the funeral director. Why not bury the aged veteran and get out of the cold? But they hesitated. Just before the announced service time, an elderly gentleman walked into the tent and sat down. After concluding a brief ritual, Reverend Nelson walked over to the sole mourner. 'Mr. President, why are you here? It's cold and bitter. Did you know this gentleman?' Harry S. Truman looked at the casket of a World War I comrade and replied, 'Pastor, I never forget a friend.'"*
>
> *David McCullough (1992, p. 985)*

One can only imagine what might have happened if Reverend Nelson had proceeded prior to the announced service time and President Truman *had* arrived to find his friend already buried. This story illustrates several points. First, whether a funeral is large or small is a non-issue. Even one mourner is of profound importance. Second, the time of impending death and its aftermath is a golden opportunity to provide outstanding leadership and be a pastoral care giver in the truest sense. In this instance and in countless millions of others, pastoral care is about ministry to the bereaving. What it is primarily not, though, is about having answers: Trying to "fix things." Alternatively, pastoral care is about the following:

- being available
- being approachable
- being interruptible
- being teachable
- being knowledgeable
- being prepared.

One of the ways in which one can be better prepared is to have self-understanding about the effects, influences, and feelings of personal losses experienced. Such understanding can be facilitated by working through the following "Personal Loss History" developed by Nancy Crump.

Personal Loss History

BIRTH _____ NOW

Starting with your birth, place a perpendicular line through your "life" line to represent loss or death in your life. After completing your loss history, answer some of the following questions about each loss.

- How do you remember reacting to the news of the loss?
- How do you remember feeling about the loss?
- How did others react to you (with silence, no support)?
- What kind of coping skills did you use?
- What made you feel better?
- What made you feel worse?
- How did this loss affect your life at the time?
- How does this loss affect your life today?

"Feed manna to hungry people. Providing information about end-of-life issues improves the quality of life for all involved with the dying."

SLJ

Two dominant themes run throughout the pages of this book: "difference making" and "making special." As a pastoral care giver at a most critical time in people's lives:

- you can make a difference in, and make special, the lives of dying individuals
- you can make a difference in, and make special, the lives of the bereaved
- you can give individuals permission to grieve
- you will have opportunities to encourage people to grieve thoroughly
- you will have opportunities to counsel people to give grief its voice
- you will have opportunities to witness, with fond admiration, the grief pilgrimages of brave, courageous individuals.

"The tender, quiet, heavily weighted moments of ministering to people amid death may prove to be among the most meaningful events of a year's work (even of a lifetime of work), those most often dreamed about, those remembered years later, those that best offer opportunities to mediate God's love to human brokenness, those that infuse the rest of ministry with profound inconspicuous significance."

Thomas Oden (1983, p. 296)

Finally, dying, death and bereavement are platinum moments for pastoral care. Therefore, as one who desires to become articulate in or train others in the artistry of pastoral care, utilize this resource unto that end. We believe that you can:

Make a difference! Make special!

Note

Statements directly attributable to a particular author will be identified by the designation of SLJ for Steven L. Jeffers and HIS for Harold Ivan Smith.

Spirituality is like a river flowing through every person.
Unfortunately, it can be dammed
in times of illness, dying,
or bereavement with
pain, fear, and loneliness.
However, a compassionate,
caring presence can prevent
the dam from forming and
keep the river flowing.

Steven L. Jeffers

Pastoral Care: Grounded in Being

"No. I'm doing okay. Thank you for coming." Have you ever heard those or similar words when attempting to offer your support to a person or persons in a time of crisis which involved death? Moreover, have you responded similarly to someone making overtures of support to you and your family at a period when one of your loved ones was dying or dead? The answer to both of those questions is, most likely, **yes**. Why is that so? Was it because we were, or at least felt, truly "okay?" Was it because we were offended by the one seeking to administer pastoral care for any number of reasons: feeling patronized with platitudes; feeling that the "intruder" was condescending? Was it because we simply wanted to be alone at that moment? Once again, the answer to those three questions in any number of scenarios is unequivocally **yes**. However, there is another reason why some people reject pastoral care, even in these times of great distress—humiliation. Well-known theologian Paul Tillich states the following:

> "When I hear the term pastoral care, I sometimes imagine myself to be in the situation of receiving pastoral care, and imagining this, I somehow feel humiliated. Someone else makes me an object of his care, but no one wants to be an object, and therefore, he resists such situations like pastoral care."
>
> *Paul Tillich (1959)*

This line of thought is quite provocative. Tillich, though, has more to say on this subject.

> "Is this feeling of resistance a necessary concomitant of pastoral care? Perhaps it cannot be removed completely, but it can be reduced to a great extent. There are two reasons for this possibility. The first is that care, including pastoral care, is something universally human. It is going on always in every moment of human existence. The second more important reason is that care is essentially mutual: he who gives care receives care. In most acts of taking care of someone, it is possible for the person who is the object of care also to become a subject."
>
> *Paul Tillich (1959)*

Can the "helpee" become the helper? Is it possible that such a role reversal may occur? Tillich says, yes.

> "Care is universally human. No one can take care of himself in every respect ... We cannot develop healthily unless we find the power of being which we lack in the power of being of others who have it, and whom we can let participate in our power of being. This encounter can be in words, and it can be in silence. From this it follows that we are taken care of if we take care of others. It is one act and not two, and only because it is one act is real care possible ... All of this is valid for pastoral care."
>
> *Paul Tillich (1959)*

The operative phrase in Tillich's words that reflects the overall message of this book is "*... we are taken care of if we take care of others.*" As pastoral care givers, we do not stand on the outside looking in. On the contrary, one who properly offers pastoral care is on the inside experiencing the pain, suffering, and healing with the objects of his care. In this sense, a pastoral care giver is subject as well as object.

In these first few pages and even in the book's title, a two-word phrase appears repeatedly: *pastoral care.* What, if anything, distinguishes pastoral care from other types of care: psychotherapy, for example? According to Tillich, the single distinguishing characteristic of pastoral care from all other forms of care is that the answer to the human situation is the divine revelation. Thus, pastoral care is "*genuine theological work.*"

> *"At the end of life, people are more spiritual than physical or mental."*
>
> *SLJ*

In a paper entitled "Creative Ministry" (2000), Clinical Pastoral Education (CPE) Supervisor Ed Outlaw pointedly addresses this distinction. Outlaw suggests that a pastoral care ministry is delineated from other caring ministries by the presuppositions and attitudes required. Several of these are poignant for this discussion.

- **Intentionality:** A pastoral care provider intentionally has a presence as representative of God who is a healer and redeemer. This understanding of the Divine Being is reflected in and experienced by faith communities through a variety of means—sacred literature, liturgy and ritual.
- **Compassion:** While not unique to pastoral care, compassion does come more acutely into focus when expressions of care for others are based upon the supposition that people are children of God.
- **Faith:** A personal faith in God (whatever one's religious tradition may be) is necessary to communicate effectively God's love and concern for people. Furthermore, individuals cannot credibly relate to God's caring presence unless such is part of their own experience.

Subsequent to the discussion on presuppositions and attitudes, Outlaw relates that an effective pastoral care giver must possess theological, philosophical, and technical knowledge.

- **Theological/God:** Knowledge of God with respect to attributes and characteristics is paramount. (As Tillich stated, this is the defining mark of care as pastoral.) These include things related to God's nature as holy, transcendent/immanent, loving, etc. Added to this would be theological knowledge of "salvation," which is spoken of in various faith traditions—Judaism, Islam, Hinduism, Buddhism, and Christianity—although the nomenclature may differ. A theological understanding of God and dying/death is essential for grief ministry.
- **Philosophical/Humanity:** Knowledge of anthropology and the humanities is also helpful in pastoral care. Human finiteness in contrast to the divine infinite, human frailty, issues of suffering, pain, illness, dying/death, and the enigma of theodicy are key issues of concern, especially in dealing with the bereaved. Humans as tripartite beings—mind, body, spirit—is also an important distinction to keep in mind. Added to these is a concern of soul immortality (understood differently among the world's major religions). There are other things as well,

such as humans as social, sexual, independent/dependent, gender-specific, religious beings with unique stories.

- **Technical/Setting:** Ministry takes place in varied settings.
  - Institutional: This would be most likely a healthcare or residential care facility, or prison/jail. Knowledge of the specified institution concerning standards of conduct, procedures, etc. is most helpful. The more informed one is with said policies, and the more one honors those policies, the more welcome he or she will be to minister in that setting. "Ecumenism" (i.e. an openness to and respect of differing faith traditions) is an important consideration in these settings.
  - Ecclesiastical: By definition, this implies that the setting would be a parish, temple, church, synagogue, or mosque. Once again, policies, traditions, and procedures are important for the pastoral care giver to know. Theological issues will also be an area of concern for ministry in a religious setting.
  - Secular: This is an umbrella term utilized to incorporate any setting not covered by institutional and ecclesiastical. Business and industry, government, and the military are examples of secular settings. Of utmost importance in secular settings would be a working knowledge of human relations with particular reference to labor and management issues. "Ecumenism" is also important in secular settings.

However, this body of knowledge and even the correct attitudes are not sufficient for highly effective pastoral care to happen. Certain skills are essential: communication (oral and written), perceptive listening and the ability to facilitate helping people identify and say what they feel, fear, and need.

Furthermore, effective pastoral care includes intuitiveness, creativity, innovation, training, and, foremost, passion and desire to help people overcome difficult circumstances and, in Tillich's words, achieve "fulfillment of human potentialities" (Tillich, 1959). He goes on to say that the all-embracing aim of pastoral care is acceptance: self-acceptance.

> "Acceptance of one's existential predicament of being finite, estranged by guilt, confronted by doubt can only be overcome by the power of the divine. Pastoral care leads to self-acceptance in spite of the ambiguity of one's being."
>
> Paul Tillich (1959)

This statement has profound significance for those who offer pastoral care in dying and death situations, for it is in those scenarios where one's finiteness (i.e. mortality), guilt and doubt (ambiguity, second-guessing) surface in acuity.

Finally, does a person have to be a great personality, a great theologian, highly educated, a great orator, and an ordained clergy person to be a pastoral care giver? Tillich says not, and we concur with that assessment.

> "The power of the divine spirit, which alone makes successful pastoral care possible, transcends the personal existence of the counselor."
>
> Paul Tillich (1959)

Let us offer one final word of counsel on the ministry of pastoral care before we proceed with discussions of other pastoral care related concerns: differing types of grief and ministry to various groups of people. One very important thing in pastoral care is the correct use of religious language. We agree with Tillich that:

> *"... we must be careful that people whom we want to help by pastoral care are not repelled, from the very beginning, by the words and symbols we use. The problem of communication is one of the greatest and most difficult in present day religious life, especially in pastoral care."*
>
> *Paul Tillich (1959)*

It is best, in many instances, to speak directly in words which convey the realities we want to share and to acknowledge openly the struggle wherein words do not seem to fit the vastness of the topic.

In short, be careful what you say, while at the same time be sensitive to the needs of the people to whom you provide care.

What should be the agenda for pastoral care? **It is the fulfillment of the needs of those in crisis, not to address issues of the care giver.** Pastoral care is a helping encounter in the dimension of ultimate concern.

> *"The ministry of a person with a heart of compassion for helping people in crisis is far more effective than a person highly skilled and trained in pastoral care but who views the role as simply a job."*
>
> *SLJ*

2

A Ministry of Presence with the Bereaved

"I believe in being fully present ... that means you should be with the person you're with."
Morrie Schwartz in Tuesdays with Morrie (Albom, 1997, p. 135)

Bereavement offers exceptional "windows" of opportunity for spiritual impact and care. Faith matters are often seen in a whole new perspective and with a new intensity under the crushing weight of grief. When one can no longer say, "It cannot happen to *me*," this fresh awareness of vulnerability and powerlessness offers incredible occasions for spiritual growth to which the pastoral care giver must respond.

What, though, does a care giver say or do in those awkward moments of life when the scent of death is everywhere, when the reality of such is pierced by wailing or silent shock? One thing is certain; ministry to the bereaved cannot be learned in an academic setting. Similarly, sensitivity cannot be learned from reading a book— even this book.

"Only by being there as the one who ... is shepherd of souls in the presence of death do we learn what to say, in part, by listening to what is being said. If we let the person tell us where he or she is, we will soon learn how best to respond."
Thomas Oden (1983, p. 299)

Pastoral care is increasingly learned in the laboratory of life using the method of "action and reflection." I (SLJ) remember an incident in our Emergency Department involving a baby. After working for a considerable length of time, the medical team was unable to revive the unconscious child. Needless to say, emotions were high for all involved: family, doctors, nurses, specialty technicians and me.

Following the passage of time and some debriefing with the Emergency Department personnel, I approached one of the treating physicians and we embraced each other. Then I said: "Doc, they didn't teach you anything about this in medical school, did they?" Without saying a word, he shook his head, implying "No!" My response to that was, "They didn't teach me anything about this in seminary either." Upon reflection of that horrific experience, I remember that I *said* very little. What I *did*, though, was by far more meaningful and helpful; I provided a shoulder and open arms by simply "being present."

"When does end of life begin? It begins at birth. Therefore, those who provide care for the dying and loved ones should take a position as ones who themselves are humbly impermanent."
SLJ

Conversely, pastoral care givers can say the right things, read the appropriate sacred literature, recite the correct prayer for the moment and still fail. Why do they fail when they do everything "by the book?" It is because they do not allow themselves to be deeply moved by *this* death. Thus, ministry with the dying and grieving must never be routine. You may have ministered in scores, or even hundreds, of cases involving dying and death. However, for someone, *this* is her elderly mother, and it is the first time she has ever lost a loved one. Still, some may have experienced other deaths, but this one is different.

> *"Death is a regular occurrence in daily life. However, each death is unique."*
>
> SLJ

Even though pastoral care has a rich, storied, timeless tradition, it is in the multiple, repetitive, timely moments of each unique death wherein the care giver has opportune occasions for making a difference in people's lives. In those circumstances of extreme adversity, there are at least four things grievers desperately want from a pastoral care provider:

1. presence with the dying and/or grieving person
2. competence in the art and science of care giving
3. sensitivity to the person's feelings and emotions
4. awareness of any underlying issues.

Furthermore, the ability to grieve in a healthy manner will often be influenced by at least three things:

1. the quality of the pastoral care received
2. the pastoral care not received but expected
3. community and family support.

> *"Every death is a once-in-a-lifetime experience, but the subsequent grief for a missed opportunity of pastoral care may well last a lifetime."*
>
> HIS

Unfortunately, missed, or even "botched," opportunities for ministry happen. Once, though, is too often if it was your mother, child, spouse, or loved one who died. For the bereaved loved ones, this is the only death of that particular person they will ever experience. Similar to missed or botched opportunities for ministry to the grieving is what might be termed "rationed" pastoral care. Harold Ivan Smith relates an experience in which a bereaved family member stated, "Let's put it this way: the minister didn't go out of his way to help us."

This, too, is not altogether uncommon in this present fast-paced American society. In *The Effective Pastor* (1985), Robert Anderson shares this story of the pastoral care he and his family received when his father died.

> *"The public details—those things that would be noticed by the public—were done rather well. I am sure, for instance, that those attending the funeral were struck by the beauty and order of the service ... In the more private details, however, —those things pertaining to the initial and continuing needs of the grieving—both the pastor and the church would have to receive a very poor grade. Yet, the more private matters were the ones the family members considered especially important."*
>
> Robert Anderson (1985, pp. 253–254)

This scenario and others like it are not intended to be indictments against all pastoral care providers. Certainly, there are legions of stories about ministers who have gone the extra mile, who have "been there" for grieving families at the time of death and long afterwards. However, Anderson's experience does highlight these poignant words of Richard Dobbins:

> *"When the funeral is over, your pastoral work is just beginning."*
> *Richard Dobbins (2000, p. 71)*

Dobbins' words punctuate the need for "aftercare" programs in faith communities, hospitals, hospices, nursing homes and funeral homes.

In this era of rationed or minimal pastoral care, there is an increasing number of people who receive no or, at best, poor pastoral care:

- those who are very affluent
- those with mental and emotional disorders
- those marginalized by society
- those of highly dysfunctional families
- those not involved in a faith congregation
- those not conversant in English
- those without a home
- those involved in ministry to suffering humanity:
  - attorneys
  - financial planners
  - executives
  - pastoral care providers
  - healthcare professionals
- those who identify themselves as atheists or agnostics
- those whose loved one died in another locale.

This last point brings into focus "there versus here" encounters with death and pastoral care. Given the mobility of society, such experiences are becoming commonplace. Consider the story of Jan, member of a faith congregation in Overland Park, Kansas. When her father died, Jan immediately returned to her home in West Virginia for the funeral. Her church in Kansas did send flowers for the funeral. After Jan returned to Overland Park, all she received in bereavement care was one note from a congregational associate minister. Consequently, Jan felt "let down" and unsupported by her faith congregation, concluding, "I expected more."

This story does not reflect all, or even the majority of, "there versus here" experiences. But it does happen, and all too frequently. Because of such, the "Jans" in religious communities will evaluate both their own experiences and their expectations with respect to pastoral care. For some of those people, the lack of pastoral care becomes one or more of the following:

- motivation to change faith congregations, maybe even change religions
- source of festering discontent: "My faith community failed me"
- unfortunate incident reflecting: "That's the way things are these days"
- indictment against all clergy and religion in general
- feelings of "I do not deserve any better care."

In this hectic world when extra time is a precious, rare commodity, those who attempt to comfort the bereaved should reflect on these words:

> *"When the care giver is an active, rather than occasional, companion who walks alongside grieving individuals, many will overlook all manner of homiletical or personal inadequacies in one who is, in deed, in crisis, a pastoral care giver."*
>
> *HIS*
>
> *"It is a rare and distinct privilege of ministry to be welcomed into the small, quiet, broken circle of the family in such critical times."*
>
> *"Two life moments are unparalleled in awakening a sense of awe: beholding a birth, and standing in the presence of death."*
>
> *Thomas Oden (1983, p. 293)*

Oden's words suggest that the pastoral care giver is called to be a guest and a witness in the life crises of others.

In conclusion, we think the importance of adequate pastoral care for the grief-stricken has been amply stated. Pastoral care, even in this time-compressed world, must never become a "fast-food drive-thru" or "microwave" endeavor. We are not dealing here with "grief lite." On the contrary, of infinite value, worth and necessity are pastoral care givers who do offer compassionate care of the soul.

Those of you who take the time to care for the dying and bereaved perform an invaluable service. The importance of such work is reflected in the words of Howard Clinebell, Jr.:

> *"Ministers occupy a central and strategic role as counselors in our society ... on the front lines in the struggle to lift the loads of troubled persons."*
>
> *Howard Clinebell, Jr. (1966/1984, p. 49)*

3

Grief: An Anthology

Humans respond to any loss through a process called grief. According to *Dorland's Illustrated Medical Dictionary* (1994, p.771), grief is defined as *"the normal emotional response to an external and consciously recognized loss."* We would like to expand that definition: *"Grief is the normal emotional, spiritual, physical, relational, financial, professional, mental response to an external and consciously recognized loss."* The addition of the extra words makes the definition consistent with the belief that healing is holistic in nature. It is a well-known fact that grief-stricken people not only suffer emotionally but in other aspects of their lives as well. Therefore, to ensure healthy grieving, appropriate ministerial strategies must consider assessment and treatment of these various components of what it means to be human.

Unfortunately, a lot of work still needs to be done in the promotion of healthy grieving, which takes time. The following observation by Victoria Alexander in *Words I Never Thought To Speak: Stories of Life in the Wake of Suicide* (1991) confirms the previous statement.

> *"Our society has little tolerance for grief. We expect it to be discreet, tidy, and above all, short-lived. Memorial services, burials, wakes … are appointed occasions for expressing loss and grief. Once these rites have been completed, the survivors are supposed to grieve privately and be done with it as quickly as possible."*
>
> *Victoria Alexander (1991, p. 159)*

All too commonly, this culture communicates that your loss does not seem too important in the grand scheme of things. "Life must go on." And that it does, leaving you **alone** in the struggle to make some sense of your overwhelming loss and to begin the healing process. This is a sad commentary on the way of life. We need a wake-up call: "Slap! Slap! 'Thanks, I needed that.'" Legions of losses every day compete for recognition and a compassionate pastoral response. At this very moment, some adolescent will experience the ending of a relationship only to hear: "She wasn't right for you anyway. You will find someone else." Similarly, two young parents will lose a baby at birth. In feeble attempts to provide comfort, people will say: "At least you have other children" or "You can have another one." As you are reading this, some middle-aged worker is being terminated because of corporate restructuring or downsizing. Typical responses would be something like this: "You can find another job," "God never closes one door without opening another," or "You were too good for them anyway." Were those adequate, compassionate responses to the individuals experiencing the losses described? We think not.

In the following pages, we will discuss differing types of grief people experience along with strategies for appropriate pastoral responses. Before we proceed, take a moment and write down some of the losses you have experienced (*see* Box 3.1).

Box 3.1   List of Losses I Have Experienced

Loss of _____	Loss of _____
Loss of _____	Loss of _____
Loss of _____	Loss of _____
Loss of _____	Loss of _____
Loss of _____	Loss of _____
Loss of _____	Loss of _____
Loss of _____	Loss of _____
Loss of _____	Loss of _____
Loss of _____	Loss of _____
Loss of _____	Loss of _____

What types of losses have you experienced? Did you cite any of these?

- Loss of a family member, loved one, or close friend by death.
- Loss of a job.
- Loss of a marriage through separation or divorce.
- Loss of a well-loved pet.
- Loss of a work colleague.
- Loss of an investment or investment opportunity.
- Loss of health.
- Loss of a special home through relocation.
- Loss of a faith community from the "way it used to be."

This list contains only a small few of the many losses people encounter throughout their lifetimes. Furthermore, each loss is accompanied by pain and suffering, which we call grief. In order for pastoral care givers to provide adequate pastoral responses to the multiplicity of losses people experience, grief specialists have developed an inventory of differing categories of grief with which care givers should become familiar:

- anniversary grief
- anticipatory grief
- delayed grief
- destructive–redemptive grief
- disenfranchised grief
- exaggerated grief
- inhibited grief
- stacked grief
- traumatic grief.

Anniversary Grief

"Often the anticipation of the anniversary is worse than the actual day."
Helen Fitzgerald (1994, p. 115)

How true those words are for so many people, especially if the anniversary of the loss is on a holiday or some other significant day in the life of a griever or grieving family. Harold Ivan Smith recounts a story from his own experience.

> *"My grandfather died on Christmas Eve. For the next thirty Christmas Eves, my mother would say, 'Well, I guess you remember what happened x number of years ago today.' Anniversary grief was troublesome because it was linked to the holidays. If my grandfather had died on July 18 or September 19, that would not have been as memorable ..."*
>
> *HIS*

What should the anniversary of a significant loss be: a time to remember, reflect, respect, and reconcile? One of the greatest fears people have about dying is that they will be forgotten. Paying attention to anniversaries prohibits this from happening. On those special days, we remember, reflect vividly and graphically on that person's life with us, and pay our respects to them. What are some of those red-letter anniversaries other than holidays?

- Birthdays.
- Wedding anniversaries.
- Special anniversaries (first date, first home, retirement, etc.)
- Death anniversaries.

Unfortunately, many grievers have to be clandestine about honoring or remembering the anniversary, sometimes even with family and friends, because our culture discourages this particular type of grief with its insistence on "getting over it and moving on." Then, there are those anniversaries that we would like to get over and move beyond, but we cannot. We are speaking of anniversaries of gruesome, horrific events: the crash of a bus, train or plane that killed scores or hundreds of people; the mass murder of innocent people such as the incident at Columbine High School in a suburb of Denver, the bombing of the Murrah Federal Building in Oklahoma City, or the events of September 11, 2001, which catapulted the United States and her allies into a global war against terrorism.

Interestingly, according to an article in *Time* magazine in December 1999, A. Goldstein relates that Frank DeAngelis, principal of Columbine High School, had April 20, 1999, permanently imbedded in his mind and in his soul. How could he ever forget that fateful day when two students went on a shooting rampage, brutally executing eleven people (ten students and one teacher) and then killing themselves? How will the city of Denver, the state of Colorado, or these United States ever forget? Yet, anticipating the first anniversary of that tragedy on April 20, 2000, he organized a committee to ensure that the anniversary was a memorial rather than a flashback. Unquestionably, DeAngelis was attempting to facilitate a means for healing in a manner similar to that described in Anne Brener's *Mourning and Mitzvah: A Guided Journal for Walking the Mourner's Path Through Grief to Healing* (1993):

> *"Giving ourselves time to heal and creating space for the process allows the painful memories to be replaced gradually by more pleasant ones. The pain*

subsides, and one remembers the whole relationship, not just the most recent memories of illness and death. We make peace with what is unresolved.''
Anne Brener (1993, p.148)

There are also times when anniversary grief is denied or, at least, forced below the surface of conscious acknowledgment. This can happen when an individual has remarried after the death of a spouse, particularly if the new marriage was premature, and perhaps to avoid doing grief work. In cases like these, widowed people want the past to be the past. If any grief work is done, it will be done by those family members or friends with whom the loss was shared or in the corridors of one's own memory. Thus, a teen-aged or young adult child may feel ambiguity with respect to anniversary grief because he or she senses that it cannot be shared with a parent who has remarried.

''The heart is the memory bank of relationships.''
SLJ

We will never forget a significant loss. Furthermore, grief repressed or denied is grief prolonged. Therefore, make special those anniversaries. In *How Will I Get Through the Holidays: 12 Ideas for Those Whose Loved One Has Died*, James Miller (1996) notes one widow's ingenuity. Every year she buys her deceased husband a cow by making a donation to the Heifer Project, which was his favorite charity.

Options for consideration by pastoral care givers to enable grievers to recognize anniversaries are:

- encourage grievers to find a way to honor the special day by making new traditions
- counsel grievers to make family and friends aware of the approaching anniversary and be willing to disclose any distress
- suggest to someone in the griever's faith community to have people in place to remember the griever on anniversaries and holidays through a phone call or sending a card.

''Be compassionate ... And take responsibility for each other. If we only learned those lessons, this world would be so much better a place.''
Morrie Schwartz in Tuesdays with Morrie (Albom, 1997, p. 163)

Anticipatory Grief

Which is more devastating to grievers: to know that death is imminent with time for preparation and to say good-byes or when death comes as a complete surprise, an ambush? Many would confirm that death as complete surprise is more severe. In fact, that has been our experience through the years as pastoral care givers. What is it that lessens the punch of death in the former scenario? The answer to that question is anticipatory grief. Helen Fitzgerald in *The Mourning Handbook* describes an event in her own life:

''I used the time during my husband's dying to express and feel my grief. I had a chance to live a life without him even though he was still alive and, most important, I had a chance to say goodbye and put closure on our relationship. I also had an opportunity to begin rebuilding my life without him before he died.''
Helen Fitzgerald (1994, p. 55)

After reflecting upon these words, I (SLJ) can relate Fitzgerald's experience to that of my family and me during the dying process of my father.

For many, anticipatory grief begins with a diagnosis: "It's *cancer,*" the most frightening phrase in the English language for many people. When such occurs, people are so overwhelmed that they are unable to see or hear any measure of hope. "My life is over. How can I live without him?" Hello! He is not dead *yet.* While a terminal diagnosis does radically alter people's lives to the point that they will never be the same, life can still be good. The last chapter of a person's life can be the absolute best for him or her and other family members.

I am reminded of the words of Dr. William Bartholome, a pediatrician and professor of medicine as well as a bioethics pioneer, who penned his "Seven Lessons on Dying" while he himself was dying. The first of those lessons is:

> *"People who are dying live in the present."*
>
> *Dr. William Bartholome*

Bartholome relates in a videotaped interview, filmed only months before his death in 1999 after being diagnosed as terminal in 1995, that his life was so fulfilled following the diagnosis he would not want to live without being considered as terminal. When something or someone takes away your future, all you have left is the present. Dr. Bartholome lived *and* grieved at the same time; he enjoyed life and prepared for death. Anticipatory grief enabled him and his family to enjoy their time together, complete unfinished business and have no regrets.

> *"The best way to live today is to prepare for tomorrow. To live life at its fullest, one must be prepared to die."*
>
> *SLJ*

To many dying individuals, life becomes more precious. Addressing any unfinished business, regrets and reconciling any estrangement in relationships are paramount. They are proactive in relationship completion using the five steps described by pioneer hospice physician Ira Byock in *The Four Things That Matter Most: A Book about Living*:

1. "I forgive you."
2. "You forgive me."
3. "I love you."
4. "Thank you."
5. "Good-bye."

After the diagnosis—or in anticipation of the diagnosis—a pastoral care giver may be summoned by family members. In one setting, individuals may want the care giver—as a representative of God—to hear, join in or even lead the "bargaining." He or she may also need to help the grievers process the "anger and denial" which have created distance in the relationship with the dying person and, thus, facilitate reconciliation. In another setting, people may solicit the pastoral figure to talk their loved one out of wanting to die and encourage him or her to keep on fighting, or to pursue other treatment. In this case, the care giver acts as a mediator by enabling honest, even painful, communication to take place. He or she can also help family members understand that "giving in" is not "giving up." It is simply a peaceful "letting go" in order that what time is left might be meaningful and productive.

"Death is vicious; Death is gift.
Death is sorrow; Death is joy.
Death is hanging on; Death is letting go."
                    Valerie Yancey *(Conference speech; 24 September 1999)*

In the previous paragraph, the words bargaining, anger, and denial are descriptors of grief popularized by Elisabeth Kubler-Ross, MD, in the 1960s—a theme to be explored in Chapter 9 entitled "Stages of Grief: Fact or Fiction?" One limiting factor of using the Kubler-Ross model is its focus on the present state (i.e. the process of dying).

Therese Rando has broadened the understanding of anticipatory grief to include past, present and future losses.

> *"Anticipatory mourning is the phenomenon encompassing seven generic oper-*
> *ations (grief and mourning, coping, interaction, psychosocial reorganization,*
> *planning, balancing conflicting demands, and facilitating an appropriate death)*
> *that, in oneself or a significant other are the recognition of associated losses in the*
> *past, present and future."*
>
>   Therese Rando *(2002, 2 May).*

Rando expanded the initial concept of anticipatory grief in several significant ways. She viewed it as a multidimensional concept defined across two perspectives, three time foci, and three classes of influencing variables. Anticipatory grief is not confined to the experience of the care giver or family alone: the dying patient also experiences this grief. In addition, Rando considered anticipatory grief to be a misnomer suggesting that one is grieving solely for anticipated losses.

Rando suggested that there are three foci of losses that occur as part of the anticipated grief: *past losses* in terms of lost opportunities and past experiences that will not be repeated; *present losses* in terms of the progressive deterioration of the terminally ill person, the uncertainty, and the loss of control; and *future losses* that will ensue as a consequence of the death, such as economic uncertainty, loneliness, altered lifestyle, and the day-to-day moments in life that will no longer occur because of death. Variables influencing anticipatory grief, according to Rando, include: *psychological factors*—the nature and meaning of the loss experienced; *social factors*—those dimensions within the family and socioeconomic characteristics that allow for certain comforts and discomforts during the illness period; and *physio-logical factors*—the griever's energy and overall health (Joan Beder, www.death reference.com/Gi-Ho/Grief.html, "Anticipatory").

Rando's more current work on anticipatory grief (*Clinical Dimensions of Anticipatory Mourning: Theory and Practice in Working with the Dying, Their Loved Ones and Their Caregivers*, 2000) broadens the work she did in the mid-1980s. This book critically examines the experience of anticipatory mourning in life-threatening and terminal illness from the perspectives of the life-threatened or dying person, their loved ones, and their care givers. There is novel incorporation into anticipatory mourning of the clinical concepts regarding coping, traumatic stress, tasks of dying, transitions to coping in absence, fading away, appropriate death, therapeutic denial, and the re-creation of meaning in illness, among many other topics. Specifically, practical intervention strategies are offered with emphasis placed on clinically relevant intervention techniques to enable healthy anticipatory mourning. We highly recommend this resource as a valuable tool in caring for people experiencing anticipatory grief.

However, we would add one more category to her list of psychological, social, and physiological factors—*spiritual factors* (the primary subject matter of this book). Among some religious people of certain faith traditions, a diagnosis has prompted an intense spiritual battle in which family, friends, colleagues, even strangers are enlisted to pray on a regular basis for physical healing. If some express skepticism or doubt concerning the restoration of health, they are ridiculed and criticized for their perceived lack of faith and may be denied access to the patient. By not unequivocally expecting complete physical healing, they are believed to be working against the best interests of the patient by not fully believing in and expecting God to perform a miracle of healing. In cases like this, the pastoral care giver may be asked and expected to pray for healing.

I (SLJ) recall an instance when I was summoned to the Emergency Department. Upon arrival, I found a young woman in her mid-thirties with a broken leg. She had requested that a chaplain come and pray with her. However, she proceeded to tell me what to pray for and how to word the prayer. I was to pray that God would heal her broken leg without surgery because her husband had broken a leg some months previously, and surgery was unnecessary for his situation. After visiting with her for awhile, I prayed that her leg be healed, without surgery if possible. Additionally, I told God that we would leave the method for healing up to Him as He worked through and guided the medical team caring for her. If surgery was the best means for healing, that would be acceptable. Following the prayer, I could tell she was deeply moved and appreciative of the prayer and the time we shared.

As pastoral care givers, be careful how you respond to patient requests. By doing as asked, you might cause more harm than good: if healing does not occur, it is your and/or God's fault. Pastoral care givers might do well to have and subscribe to their own Hippocratic oath.

"First, do no harm."

HIS

Perhaps the most important thing that a pastoral care giver can do in seasons of anticipatory grief is to listen—listen to the narratives of patients and their families. The Amish have a wonderful saying: "Listen much, talk little." Listen to what is said and to what is *not* said. Admittedly, this is something you might have to facilitate and "make happen." How healing it is to share those stories and be transparent! Such allows the patient to experience a peaceful death and the survivors to have no regrets or unfinished business. I (SLJ) spent several hours at the bedside of a dying woman with her family. Upon my arrival, I was asked to pray. I might note that my prayer was not one for physical healing but of committal of the patient into the presence of God. Shortly thereafter, as I facilitated the sharing of stories, I asked each family member (only if they were comfortable doing so) to relate that which was most memorable concerning the patient. Out of the hushed silence, one spoke and that was followed by others sharing their stories. We continued sharing through the hours until she died. Many of the family members hugged and thanked me for helping to make a most difficult time easier to bear.

Similarly, there are times when the patient is alert and family members are too distraught to listen to their loved one's words of dying and, thus, they keep busy as a way of dealing with anticipatory grief. So, the words of the patient fall upon "deaf ears." In his book *The Wisdom of Dying: Practices for Living* (1999), hospice physician Michael Murphy argues that what many patients want are individuals to witness lovingly their dying. They do not want to grapple with death alone.

> *"We have not learned that there are times, much more frequent than we imagine, when the storyteller is seeking only a witness—a human being rather than a human doing."*
>
> Michael Murphy (1999, p. 35)

The pastoral care giver can be that human *being* the faithful witness. In *The Journey Through Grief* (1997a), Alan Wolfelt of the Center for Grief and Loss Transition summarized his experience as a witness to his father's dying.

> *"As he shifted from topic to topic, he did not need me to get in the way. As he occasionally struggled with a detail of a long-ago memory, he did not need me to get in the way. As he was brought to tears by his love-filled memories of life and living, he did not need me to get in the way."*
>
> Alan Wolfelt (1997a, p. 1)

There are others like Bartholome who desire to be embraced at the end of life by a loving and supportive family. However, the key people in the diagnosed person's life may well begin heavy grieving, even to the point of distancing themselves from their dying loved one. The emotions they may express include:

- **Denial:** "This *cannot* be true" or "I don't believe this is happening."
- **Anger:** "How could you do this to me?" or "I hate you for this."
- **Bargaining:** Making promises to God seeking a divine "override" of the diagnosis: "If you will heal my husband, I will ..."

These emotional responses are normal and even expected. There is something very human about anger and denial of things considered unpleasant, such as the impending death of a loved one or of bargaining to "buy a little more time" to spend with that special someone.

Conversely, there are times when terminal patients want to die and are prepared to do so. They perceive the diagnosis as a blessing, as a time to do some or all of the following things:

- say last good-byes
- work through a "to do" list
- express "memorialization" preferences
- "savor the slices of life"
- let go.

> *"Don't let go too soon, but don't hang on too long."*
> Morrie Schwartz in *Tuesdays with Morrie* (Albom, 1997, p. 162)

However, some family members or friends cannot and will not "let go." Whenever the patient broaches the subject of issues related to "letting go," the moment is sabotaged by, "Oh, now let's not talk that way" or "God is still in control, we must not give up." So, there is the insistence on trying yet another procedure, seeing another specialist or changing the subject, all of which is a total disregard for the patient's wishes.

Concerning the prevalence of complicated mourning, Therese Rando identifies "the gifts" of anticipatory grief (1984, p. 37):

- privilege of absorbing the reality of the loss gradually over time
- opportunity to take care of any unfinished business with the dying person by expressing feelings and resolving past conflicts
- chance of beginning to confront assumptions about life, one's identity, friends, God
- unhurried state of mind in making plans for the future, including the funeral rituals.

In conclusion, anticipatory grief is often unacknowledged by family members of the dying as well as pastoral care givers. It needs to be acknowledged, admitted, and addressed. We have discussed a number of issues for pastoral care givers in identifying and responding to anticipatory grief. We offer these, in addition, as suggested by Rando (1984) and Fulton and Fulton (1971).

- Anticipatory grief that resembles a roller-coaster effect leads to emotional, physical, and spiritual exhaustion. Often, individuals will begin praying that their loved ones will die soon so that their pain and suffering will cease. Such prayers can produce guilt, albeit self-inflicted. Pastoral care givers may need to hear these confessions and to assure those people that guilt for praying in that manner is natural; it is appropriate to pray in that way when someone is suffering intolerable pain and relief will only come in death.
- When a patient is expected to die and the family members are reconciled with that fact, a remission, or repeated remissions (often called the "Lazarus Syndrome"), may make it difficult for those family members to re-invest in the next and/or subsequent remission episodes. Over time, family members or close friends may feel anger, frustration, even resentment when travel, expense, and time involved cause their lives to be in constant turmoil. A pastoral care giver should be aware of such issues and the feelings that might accompany them in order that he or she can help individuals process those feelings, and most especially the strong feeling of guilt that often arises in response to the other emotions.
- Because so much attention and energy has been given to grieving before the death, loved ones may feel little need for formal closure rituals such as the funeral. However, this mindset eliminates, in Rando's words, *"an opportunity to experience the social confirmation and support such rituals afford"* (1984, p. 39). As a care giver, you are obliged to remind grievers of this necessity and actively encourage some type of ritual. Furthermore, it is in ritualizing that the finality of the death is brought clearly into focus and, thus, facilitates the thinking that "we must move forward rather than on."

Finally, pastoral care givers, while caring for the family and friends, must also pay attention to their own anticipatory grief. When you are dealing with grief—past, present, and future—in multitudes of instances simultaneously, how much is too much? One pastoral care giver said, *"I live with so much grief that some mornings I want to say, 'Okay, God, who's next? Give me a hint.'"* Such an admission is healthy. We offer you one word of counsel:

> *"Take care of yourself in order that you can more adequately care for others."*
>
> SLJ

One of the best admonitions a pastoral care giver can offer to an individual in anticipatory grief is eloquently articulated in these words.

"Give your grief its voice! Find ways to embrace that grief."

HIS

Delayed Grief

"When your loved one died, you may have taken a deep breath, put your grief on hold, and stepped forward to make the arrangements, decide on the legal matters, be executor of the will, comfort the bereaved, and generally take charge. You may even have thought that you could bypass grief by doing all of this."
Helen Fitzgerald (1994, p. 169)

These words of Fitzgerald are ample testimony to the fact that, in a time-is-money, hurry-up-and-get-over-it culture, who has time to do quality, thorough grief work? However, sooner or later, grief will get your attention, your full individual attention. Furthermore, by that later point in time, the grief may well be like compound interest on a loan (i.e. greatly increased). In this sense, grief is reminiscent of the wisdom portrayed in the Fram oil filter commercial of years past.

"You can pay me now OR you can pay me later."
Fram oil filter commercial

Grief can be delayed for a variety of reasons; we will mention only a few. When a spouse, son, daughter, or other family member has been care giver over months or years of a lingering, debilitating illness, grief may be delayed by physical and emotional exhaustion. I (SLJ) feel certain that my mother was a victim of delayed grief, although the compounded impact was lessened because of anticipatory grief.

For approximately ten long years, Mom cared for her parents (my grandparents) and her husband (my father) until their deaths, all at home. This all began in 1988 with my grandfather who died in 1989 at the age of 91 with cancer. Almost simultaneously, she started caring for my grandmother who had Alzheimer's. Granny died several years later on December 22, 1993, and was buried on Christmas Eve (anniversary grief). Finally, in 1994, my dad became seriously ill and died on August 4, 1998, of Parkinson's disease. During that time, I witnessed few expressions of grief from my mother until after the death of my father. I suppose all of that delayed grief caught up with her.

A far more common type of delayed grief happens when a family member serves as executor of the estate. The delay in grief is especially pronounced and compounded when tensions arise over details of the estate. No object or amount of money is too insignificant or small to ignite a "tug-of-wills." Even without those heightened kinds of tensions, many executors feel compelled to put their grief "on hold" in order to deal with the overwhelming demands of the bureaucracy of death—a myriad of detailed forms to be completed, notarized, recorded, and filed.

The nightmare of mega proportions occurs, though, for families of individuals who died intestate—without an estate plan. The anger and frustration that erupts in such situations interferes with the grief work: "How could you have done this to us?!" My (SLJ) mother has a very wealthy first cousin who became engaged in an ongoing battle with the Inland Revenue Service (IRS) when her parents died

First published 2007 by Radcliffe Publishing

Published 2016 by CRC Press
Taylor & Francis Group
6000 Broken Sound Parkway NW, Suite 300
Boca Raton, FL 33487-2742

ISBN-13: 978-1-84619-181-7 (pbk)

Visit the Taylor & Francis Web site at
http://www.taylorandfrancis.com

and the CRC Press Web site at
http://www.crcpress.com

British Library Cataloguing in Publication Data

A catalogue record for this book is available from the British Library.

Typeset by Advance Typesetting Ltd, Oxford

Whether grief is redemptive or destructive is dependent upon the decisions made by grieving individuals. The latter can be especially true for parents who lose a child. Perhaps nothing can be more painful for a parent than to outlive a child (regardless of the child's age). If the parents grieve independently, one spouse may become involved in an affair as a way of seeking comfort the other spouse does not provide. Furthermore, and even though there is no substantiating research data to support this statement, tensions may erupt to a breaking point in the marriage resulting in a separation or divorce.

> *"I can have a pretty good day and then I get home. I don't even have to go inside to know she has been crying all day. She drags me down."*
>
> *Tom, a grieving father*

Unless Tom and his wife can communicate and share their grief, their individual grieving could result in disaster for their relationship.

Moreover, surviving siblings may feel ignored by the grieving parent and "act up" to gain attention. Siblings may also feel guilty about incidents of sibling rivalry that were unresolved, and death has taken away the possibility of reconciliation. In other cases, the marriage or the entire family relationship was on shaky ground, and the untimely death was the proverbial "straw that broke the camel's back." The result of that was destructive grief. Indeed, the pastoral care giver, even the highly trained one, may have difficulty sorting out these or any other realities when ministering to parents or entire families grieving over the death of a child.

A non-violent or natural death of a child, parent, or spouse is bad enough. However, when some family member of that intimate circle is killed in an "at-fault" accident or murdered, that is an occasion for grief to turn significantly destructive. In such cases, some families devote enormous amounts of energy attempting to make an institution or individual assume responsibility and/or be punished. In that lengthy process, often lasting for years, the survivors are consumed with seeing that justice is done: arrest, conviction, sentencing, and denying parole. Meanwhile, there is no time for grieving and the anger and frustration continue to gain momentum. Interestingly, some people believe that their grief will be over when "justice is served." In some cases, justice was not served in the eyes of the victim's loved ones and, thus, there was no closure. Colin Murray Parkes, from his book *Bereavement: Studies of Grief in Adult Life* (1972), has this to say about the journey of grief:

> *"Anything that continually allows the person to avoid or to suppress this pain can be expected to prolong the course of mourning."*
>
> *Colin Murray Parkes (1972, p. 173)*

Such a situation as previously described can be exacerbated if a family member or close friend may tire of investing the energy and withdraw from the process of seeking justice for the loved one's wrongful death. A decision like that often angers other family members who are still deeply committed to the process and can produce outbursts like: "Obviously, you didn't love him as much as we did" or "I always felt you never did really love her." How piercing to the soul are words like that! Even though uttered out of distress and anxiety, they still hurt deeply. The youngest of five siblings, following a multi-year crusade to avenge another brother's murder, withdrew from the family process citing these words:

"I feel like my brother is killed again every time there is a parole hearing. We relive the nightmare ... nothing will bring my brother back. But I cannot make others see that. It has become some kind of personal crusade for them ... He murdered my brother, but sometimes I feel like he murdered my family as well."
A grieving sibling

This young man feels like the obsession with his dead brother's murderer is, in reality, a "living murder" for his family. There are few things, if any at all, that are more destructive than murder, especially mass murder. One needs only to consider the initial and lasting effects of the Alfred P. Murrah Federal Building bombing in Oklahoma City, the second worst act of terrorism on United States soil, in which 168 people were mercilessly murdered by Timothy McVeigh. And, of course, who can ever forget the incident which, for many, causes Pearl Harbor to pale in comparison—the deliberate slaughter of over 3,000 innocent civilians on September 11, 2001, an event masterminded and funded by international terrorist Osama bin Laden. Think also of the July 7, 2005 terrorist bombings in the London public transit system that killed 52 people and injured over 700. For many of the victims' families and loved ones, the grief associated with these events is an example of destructive grief par excellence. This "revengeful" type of grief is like drinking poison every day and hoping the other person dies.

Finally, one's work performance may steadily deteriorate after a loved one's death when inadequate attention is paid to grief or when the employee turns to a "substance" for solace. As a result of substance abuse and/or poor work habits, some people voluntarily drop out of the work force, while others are terminated or, at best, disciplined. Unfortunately, many people do not take advantage of Employee Assistance Program (EAP) counseling until their work performance is adversely affected. In a good many cases of this nature, financial stress escalates as well as heightened levels of tension among family members. Conversely, there is the situation wherein people keep extremely busy, never slowing down. Men are especially at high risk for becoming post-death workaholics. Interestingly, whereas the death of the loved one might have been rather quick, like a fire consuming a building, the "death" of the griever, in terms of relationships of various kinds, may be ever so slow, similar to rising flood waters in a small town.

"Sometimes, it takes a long period of time for the grief to be disruptive. Not unlike a leak in the roof, the family 'colludes' to ignore the leak until a significant level of damage occurs."
HIS

Destructive grief devastates the lives of survivors. However, the antidote for this type of grief is redemptive grief, to which we now turn our attention.

Grief rarely, if ever, leaves people the same. Individuals either become bitter or better. In redemptive grief, people choose to say this to a loss: "You will not defeat me. Loss will not have the last word."

"It is not so much what happens to you BUT how you choose to respond or react."
Mark R. Moore to HIS

Bereaved people control their own grief. They do have choices. Many have chosen to respond positively and in a redemptive manner to incurred losses. One of the most significant and well-known acts of redemptive grief was an initiative by Candice Lightner following the death of her 12-year-old daughter, Cari, who was killed by a drunk driver. Using the media exposure of the incident and its aftermath, in 1980 Lightner launched MADD—Mothers Against Drunk Drivers. She used her loss as a means to reach out to others and to lobby for changes in driving standards, an effort that has been nothing short of a revolution. However, Joy Johnson reported that when Mrs. Lightner retired from MADD, she "fell apart." Why? She had put all of her energy into MADD and none into her personal grief work. This is clear evidence that there is no substitute for personal grieving.

Similarly, Charlotte Zwillinger's daughter, a college junior at the time, was murdered by her ex-boyfriend. When the killer only served less than 18 months of a three-to-five-year sentence, Zwillinger could not accept the injustice and, what her husband termed, "the conspiracy of silence." In fact, who could accept such an injustice? However, she chose to let her grief be redemptive as opposed to destructive. In 1978, the Zwillingers started "Parents of Murdered Children." As a result, their loss was not in vain, for through this organization, they have helped countless others who have experienced similar losses. "The Compassionate Friends" is a companion organization for parents who have lost children from any cause.

> *"If life experiences are not used, they are wasted."*
> *Charlotte Zwillinger (in Schlosser, 1997, p. 50)*

How provocative and poignant are those words which were cited in an article by Eric Schlosser, "A Grief Like No Other," in the September, 1997 issue of *The Atlantic Monthly*.

Some people, though, do not start organizations like MADD or Parents of Murdered Children as a way to redeem their losses. They finance gifts. One couple provided the resources for a children's play area, designed to resemble a zoo, as a memorial to honor the death of a young child. While the loss of that child will never be overcome or forgotten, the grief experienced has a profound redeeming quality. Because of the children who use the playground, their parents and the church members will have fond, continual memories of their "special friend." Still others make contributions to hospitals, faith congregations, community organizations and educational institutions as memorial gifts in the names of a deceased loved one. Such things can certainly be assets in changing destructive into redemptive grief.

> *"When out of the pain and suffering of our own loss we help others, we are, in reality, helping ourselves."*
>
> *SLJ*

Redemptive grievers often come to the realization that God has not comforted them so they can move on or get through it. On the contrary, He comforts them so that they can reach out to others whose "now" was their "yesterday." Out of much pain comes great compassion. Pastoral care givers can facilitate such by being available for support and, thus, serve as spiritual midwives in the transformation from destructive to redemptive grief. The following is a list of pastoral issues for consideration.

- Some individuals are in such intense pain that they are unable to respond to or even hear the help pastoral care givers want to provide. In cases of this nature, the care giver must gently deliver the message that "good can come out of this ... in time and with your cooperation."
- Pastoral care givers need to develop a referral list with both local and national phone numbers and addresses for organizations/support groups to help grievers who are trapped in the rut of destructive grief. It would be extremely useful for care givers to have personal knowledge of the various organizations and the services they provide. Additionally, it would be helpful to have a referral list of local clinicians (mental health professionals, pastoral counselors, etc.) who can be resources to individuals and family units impacted by the loss. (*See* Appendix B for a listing of national resource centers for help on various types of end-of-life issues.)
- Pastoral care givers need to be alert to individuals in a family or a social network who are actively resisting the redemptive dimension of the death. There can be a heightened level of tension among grievers when one gets mired in destructive grief, while others are actively pursuing redemptive grief.
- Pastoral care givers should be familiar with and encourage ways that individuals can "fund" redemptive grief (i.e. gifts, financial contributions, volunteering, etc. to institutions and/or organizations).

> *"Helping people see heaven in the hell and inextinguishable grace amidst the fires of suffering is pastoral care in the highest realm."*
>
> *SLJ*

Disenfranchised Grief

Our society has a variety of ways to sanction grief: The sending of cards and/or flowers; bereavement leave from the workplace; and, in general, "cutting grievers some slack" in fulfilling normal responsibilities. However, there are only certain relationships that society validates with its offer of support, and that circle is very small—immediate family only (parents, children, siblings, grandparents). Thus, the death of other individuals goes "un-validated," "un-allowed," or "disenfranchised."

Kenneth Doka (1989, p. 4) defines disenfranchised grief as a loss that cannot be: openly acknowledged, publicly mourned, and socially sanctioned. In his most recent work, Doka adds two additional categories (*Disenfranchised Grief: New Directions, Challenges and Strategies for Practice*, 2002). We now examine Doka's five categories of how grief can be "disenfranchised," extracted from an article he authored, entitled "Disenfranchised" (www.deathreference.com/Gi-Ho/Grief.html).

1. **The relationship is not recognized**. Grief may be disenfranchised in those situations in which the relationship between the bereaved and deceased is not a recognizable kin tie. The closeness of other non-kin relationships may simply be misunderstood or unappreciated. The roles of lovers, friends, neighbors, foster parents, colleagues, in-laws, step-parents and stepchildren, care givers, counselors, coworkers, and roommates (e.g. in nursing homes) may be close and long-standing, but even though these relationships are recognized, mourners may not have full opportunity publicly to grieve. At most, they might be expected to support and assist family members.

2. **The loss is not acknowledged**. In other cases, the loss is not socially recognized as significant. Individuals experience many losses—some death-related, such as perinatal loss, or other non-death-related losses such as divorce, incarceration, the loss of a job or material possessions, or significant change in personality or temperament that may be unacknowledged by others. Some losses may be intangible. For example, a teenager aspiring to a career in sports is cut from a team, or parents discover that a beloved child suffers from a disability or disease. The loss of reputation because of scandal, gossip, or arrest can be devastating. Even transitions in life can have undercurrents of loss. Aging, for example, leads to constant developmental losses such as the loss of childhood or other losses associated with different points of life.

3. **The griever is excluded**. There are situations in which the characteristics of the bereaved disenfranchise their grief. The person is not socially defined as capable of grief; therefore, there is little or no social recognition of his or her sense of loss or need to mourn. Despite evidence to the contrary, both the old and the very young are typically perceived by others as having little comprehension of or reaction to the death of a significant other. Similarly, mentally disabled persons may also be disenfranchised in grief.

4. **Circumstances of the death**. The nature of the death may constrain the solicitation of the bereaved for support and limit the support extended by others. For example, many survivors of a suicide loss often feel a sense of shame or stigma, believing that others may negatively judge the family because of the suicide. Similarly, the stigma of AIDS (acquired immune deficiency syndrome) may lead survivors of an AIDS-related loss to be cautious in sharing the loss with others.

5. **The ways an individual grieves**. The way in which an individual grieves also can contribute to disenfranchisement. Certain cultural modes of expressing grief such as stoicism or wailing may fall beyond the grieving rules of a given society, and thus contribute to disenfranchisement. Particularly is this true as diversity becomes a reality in more communities.

These categories of loss identified by Doka will be discussed variously throughout this chapter.

Unfortunately, without recognition, acknowledgement, validation of the loss for whatever the reason(s), there is often little or no support for the ones who have experienced what, for them, is a devastating loss.

"Recovery takes people. In grief, people need people."

Doug Manning (1979)

Many people have very meaningful relationships, beyond "immediate family"—aunts, uncles, cousins, nephews, nieces, friends, work colleagues. For some there is a closer bond with persons outside that small circle sanctioned by society than there is within that circle. Increasingly, individuals invest in faux families—individuals are "like" family and relationships may be more emotionally meaningful than that of blood kin.

Consider the following:

- A child is abandoned by both parents early in his life and raised by an aunt and uncle. He grew up with no feelings of closeness to his parents, even though there have been repeated attempts on the part of the parents for reconciliation.

- A young woman, estranged from her two siblings, has a long-term relationship with another individual, whom she considers dearer than a brother.
- An individual is raised by an aunt who becomes de facto parent.

What will happen when the aunt, uncle, or the person dearer than a brother dies? Will bereavement leave be available for the young man or young woman? Will they be intentionally supported? Remember, these are relationships not sanctioned by society or recognized by corporate policies on bereavement. Nevertheless, these were relationships of immense closeness, and the grievers will be crying out in words identical to the title of Manning's book: *"Don't Take My Grief Away!"* No matter how far extended a relationship may be, where there is closeness and a loss is incurred, such needs to be recognized, affirmed, and healthy grief encouraged. The skilled pastoral care giver will also hear other cries, which are applicable to any type of situation involving significant loss (*Five Cries of Grief*, Morton P. and A. Irene Strommen, 1993):

- **cry of pain**, centered in the awareness of a devastating loss
- **cry of longing**, reflecting a pervasive loneliness that results from missing the loved one
- **cry for supportive love**, arising from the extreme sense of vulnerability
- **cry for significance**, striving to see some good come out of the loss.

Doug Manning would add to this list: Finding the significance of the deceased.
 There are other types of losses which Kenneth Doka describes as "relationships not recognized" (*Disenfranchised Grief: Recognizing Hidden Sorrow*, 1989, p. 5).

> *"Nontraditional relationships, such as extramarital affairs, cohabitation, and homosexual relationships have tenuous public acceptance and limited legal standing, and they often face negative sanction within the larger community. Those involved in such relationships are touched by grief when the relationship is terminated by the death of a partner, but others in their world, such as children, may also experience a grief that cannot be acknowledged or socially supported."*
> *Kenneth Doka (1989, p. 5)*

In a culture where millions of people live in "nontraditional" relationships, significant numbers of deaths are not recognized or are *under*-recognized. Unfortunately, some deaths in those types of relationships actually set up a tug-of-war among family, lovers, and friends of the deceased.

> *"The very nature of disenfranchised grief creates additional problems for grief, while removing or minimizing sources of support."*
> *Kenneth Doka (1989, p. 4)*

Individuals in nontraditional relationships are not alone in the camp of disenfranchised grievers. Doka points to "social death" wherein a person is treated as if he or she were dead: for example, an ex-spouse. Those impacted by the broken relationship may have their grief unrecognized or even stifled by words like these: "I don't ever want to hear anyone mention his name to me again!" Or consider the ex-spouse who hears, "You're the last person I expected to be grieving after the way you were treated!" Furthermore, there are certain groups which society deems incapable of grief, at least the full understanding of the reality and magnitude of the loss. Certainly, children fall into this category as well as the mentally challenged.

Increasingly, the death of pets is often unrecognized and even disenfranchised. "It was only a dog," one man responded. "That is true," the owner countered, "but it was *my* dog!" Many pet owners have been stunned by the fact that their feelings of grief were shunned.

Finally, there are several suggestions for ministry to those whose grief is disenfranchised of which pastoral care givers need to be informed:

- Pastoral care givers must be ever mindful that a loss is a loss. It does not matter whether the relationship was traditional, nontraditional, or nonhuman. Where there was intimacy, grief occurs, and according to Dr. J. Thomas Meigs, grief is at least three things:
  1. painful
  2. necessary
  3. good.
- Pastoral care givers must recognize that grievers whose grief is not allowed or affirmed may become angry with individuals or faith communities for their lack of support. This individual may lash out at all ministers. When you encounter this hurting griever, hear out the griever without condemnation or becoming defensive.
- Pastoral care givers need to remember that, by definition, pastoral care is theological work done in the name of God who cares for the wounded.
- Pastoral care is not only about offering hospitality to the grievers but being receptive to their ideas, narratives, fears, and innovations.
- Pastoral care givers need to keep in mind that those who lack support also lack essential resources to mend. Ron DelBene relates in *A Time to Mourn: Recovering From the Death of a Loved One* (1988) that this griever must be supported, and you may be the support.

Pastoral care givers regularly counsel people to give grief its voice. Those people whose grief is disenfranchised are doing that very thing. Sadly, no one is listening. Meigs suggests that in support of those who have suffered a loss, Paul Tillich's words ought to be a guiding credo:

> *"The first duty of love is to listen."*
>
> *Paul Tillich*

Exaggerated Grief

In a culture that is "grief-lite" as well as grief-phobic, anyone doing thorough grief will be assumed to be expressing exaggerated grief. "Look at the way she is carrying on." Then comes the confrontation: "He would not want you going on like this." Harold Ivan Smith relates a stunning experience he had on a trip to London. While reading the newspaper, he found this phrase in many of the obituaries: *"No mourning."* When he called the obituary editor to ask what those two words meant, she was "taken back" and eventually sputtered: *"You know, all that crying and carrying on!"* Doug Manning has some words in his book, *Don't Take My Grief Away* (1979), as a response to that mindset:

> *"Grief is not an enemy—it is a friend. It is the natural process of walking through hurt and growing because of the walk. Let it happen. Stand up tall to*

*friends and to yourself and say, 'Don't take my grief away from me. I deserve it,
and I am going to have it.''* '

Doug Manning (1979, p. 6)

There are several things that can lead to (or at least to an assumption of) exaggerated
grief. One of these is influence of culture. For example, many Caucasians consider
grief in the African-American community to be exaggerated or excessive. In
Disenfranchised Grief: Recognizing Hidden Sorrow, by Doka, Ronald Barrett suggests
that many African-Americans do, indeed, have a much more emotional funeral
ritual than do the majority of Caucasians (Barrett, 1998). There is no sense of
shame, embarrassment, or discomfort for "venting" emotions in expressions of grief.
Manning offers that grief is encouraged and facilitated by such expressions.
Interestingly, Mitch Albom has this to say about the shame of people who are
dying—something he learned from Morrie Schwartz:

''His philosophy was that death should not be embarrassing.''

(Albom, 1997, p. 21)

Alan Wolfelt argues that the freedom to experience grief common in many African-
American funerals, and for an extended time thereafter, lessens the need for
counseling because those individuals have a socially supported, cathartic experience of mourning. On the other hand, Caucasians, generally speaking, have a small
"window of opportunity" for acceptable grief expressions: during the days of
ritualizing and the immediate subsequent days.

*''Rather than cooperating with the cultural inhibition through fears of what
people will say, think, or remember, pastoral care givers can give individuals a
wonderful gift: permission to grieve and permission to grieve thoroughly.''*

HIS

Another reason for the presence of exaggerated grief is competition among
mourners for the designation of "chief mourner." Who loved the deceased the
most? Who was the "closest?" Who did the most? Who sacrificed the most? The
theory is the one whose grief expressions were the most intense was that person. In
cases like this, grief is often linked with pre-existing rivalries, dysfunction, and/or
relational history. Suppose, for example, that a young, recently married male is
killed. Is the chief mourner (at least in the legal sense) the young man's mother or
his widow? The law would say wife, but some mothers contest such a declaration.
One such mother snapped at her daughter-in-law, "You only had him four years,
but I had him for twenty-nine years."

''Grief is not a competitive sport.''

Joy Johnson (2006)

Competition can also erupt in dysfunctional families, especially when old issues
may resurface or previous tensions are rekindled. Thus, daughters may compete
in the display of grief emotions following a father's death or the same with sons
following a mother's death. Competition in grief can also occur between family
members of blended families "yours, mine, and ours" issues.

In a grief-denying culture, many want, even demand, minimal grief and want it
kept "under control." However, the phrase "taking it hard" typifies the experience
of many grievers, often belated. This could well have been the case, at least in part,

in the public outpouring of emotion following the death of Princess Diana in 1997 as well as that of John F. Kennedy, Jr. in 1999. Many in the United States, the United Kingdom, and around the globe had grief rebooted during the ritualizing of these two famous, dynamic young adults. A lot of personal, previously unprocessed grief (delayed grief) was "unfrozen."

Several pastoral issues are important for the care giver to consider when addressing exaggerated grief, which can sometimes be understood as delayed grief "heaped" upon grief from a current incident or stacked grief (to be discussed later):

- When informed that an individual is "excessively" grieving, it is essential to ask why the expression of grief is perceived as exaggerated. Indeed, the perception may say more about the informant than the griever. In that conversation, the care giver may need to explain several things:
  - All people grieve differently.
  - What seems exaggerated grief to one individual may be quite normal and healthy.
  - Sooner or later, everyone pays the "toll" on the grief journey.
- According to an article in *The Hospice Journal* (1998) by S. B. Dowd *et al.*, multicultural responses of varied degrees of intensity happen within the same family due to intermarriage as well as friendship circles. Some immigrants, Chinese for example, consider wailing to be an indication of how much they cared for the deceased.

Be quick to listen, slow to critique.

- If the care giver decides to converse with the allegedly exaggerated griever, he or she needs to ask if there have been previous losses and how, in those instances, grief was given its voice. Of course, this conversation is not about confronting, but simply engaging in a mutually respectful dialogue.
- The astute care giver must be alert to the young person who may be experiencing his or her first significant encounter with grief, and, thus, may need some counsel on "how to grieve" healthfully.

Educating the bereaved is vitally important in order to help them "normalize" the grief journey.

Finally, additional information on differing cultural responses is needed to correct often incorrect perceptions. Pastoral care givers may find *Culture and Nursing Care: A Pocket Guide* to be an invaluable resource for offering "culturally competent" care (Lipson, 1996). This book contains insights on serious illness and death for 24 ethnic groups; it particularly calls attention to one's personal space, eye contact, touch. The authors caution care givers to remember that there is great variation among ethnic groups with respect to understanding illness, dying, and ritualizing. For example, among Hispanics, there are recent immigrants to the United States who may bring funeral customs from Mexico that are quite different from those of Puerto Rico or Brazil. Moreover, there are differences within groups shaped by social status and economics.

Do not forget these words:

> *"Excess is in the eye of the beholder. The pop song's lyric, 'You'd cry too if it happened to you' is wonderful cross-cultural advice."*

HIS

Inhibited Grief

Many people remember, all too well, the "shots heard around the world" on November 22, 1963, when President John Fitzgerald Kennedy was assassinated. Those same individuals will also recall Jackie Kennedy's public demeanor in the days following that tragedy of monumental proportion. In fact, her stoic behavior became something of a national model for grief expression, or maybe the lack thereof.

> *"A tear that is not expressed on the face seeks and find its ultimate revenge somewhere else in the body."*
>
> *Fritz Perls*

Grief specialists suggest that people who cannot "accept" the death or express their grief are inhibited. Therese Rando (1984, p. 109) has identified three factors that commonly inhibit grief:

1. dependence upon the deceased
2. fear of emotions of grief
3. guilt about the death or the relationship at the time of death.

Grief is so powerful an emotion that some individuals want to manage it, or at least confine it to a measured, controlled, private environment. For this reason, some will not cry at a funeral home or at the cemetery because they are public places; others may not cry because they think they have to get through the memorial service without "breaking down;" still others will not cry in front of certain family members and/or friends.

> *"When I was eight, my dad died unexpectedly of a heart attack. As the youngest of five siblings (four of us, boys), I looked to my brothers for guidance on how to act in this unsettling and unfamiliar territory. At Dad's funeral, I got the message. When I started crying, my brother, Mike, looked down and barked, 'Stop crying. Be a man.'"*
>
> *Kevin Jennings (1998)*

Many years hence, Jennings vividly recalls that life-changing event and shares it in an article entitled "My Perspective: Be a Man" (*The Advocate*, September 29, 1998, p. 14).

His experience supports the supposition that, traditionally, males are particularly quick to encourage strength. "Be strong" is frequently intended to be understood as an admonition, not a suggestion: "You've got to be strong for ..." or "You have to be strong to get through this" ("this" referring to the public rituals). Frequently, male grievers have confessed, "I just hope I can get through this without crying, breaking down or going to pieces." If only they could understand that crying is incredibly therapeutic; it also gives others permission to discard their inhibitions and gives an invitation for opening expressions of support and nurture. It is unfortunate that, in many families, "being strong" is expected; grieving males losing control and crying is not a pretty sight. Yet, physiologically, it is healthy.

Similarly, it is not uncommon to find inhibited grief in male-dominated professions such as police, fire, emergency response providers, and military-service personnel. In an article in the *British Journal of Criminology* (1994), Mark Burke points to a "machismo subculture," which discourages any display of tenderness or expressions of grief. (Women in these professions may be expected to grieve in the same manner as men.) Moreover, since many funerals for individuals killed in the line of duty may be large, including a significant number of "brother" comrades as well as attention of the media, publicly expressed grief may be discouraged.

> *"From working with grieving men, I have learned that the public expression of grief ... or the absence of grieving is not adequate indication of the total picture. Indeed, below the surface, can be great, grief-related stress."*
>
> *HIS*

Something of a "Titanic" effect occurs among grieving men. Like an iceberg, only 10% is visible. Our society does males—of all ages and occupations—a disservice by discouraging and limiting public expressions of their grief.

> *"It is extremely difficult for people in the caring professions to express insensitivity to a hurting humanity and, at the same time, minister effectively."*
>
> *SLJ*

Yet, inhibited grief also occurs among ministers of various faith traditions. Western, North American (i.e. United States) culture expects the professional or lay minister to remain composed regardless of the heart-wrenching details of a particular death or ritual, and they are aware of this expectation. How many times have you heard funeral or memorial service leaders make apologies—"Excuse me" or "Forgive me"—on the edge of being human (i.e. emotional)? Ministers can also inhibit others. In the movie *The Big Chill*, when the friend offering the eulogy "broke down," the minister swiftly stepped beside him and moved him away from the podium, in essence saying: "We will have no emotional displays in a funeral of which I am in charge." Interestingly, many take their cues on life, including how to express grief, from movies and television. Harold Ivan Smith relates the following story of a funeral he attended.

> *"A grandson began crying while reading his grandmother's favorite Isaiah passage. The congregation was moved to witness his tears, but not the clergy person in charge. He quickly stepped to the pulpit, whispered to the grandson who obediently sat down. Then the minister finished the reading."*
>
> *HIS*

In his book, *From the Heart: Stories of a Pastor's Walk With His People* (1991, pp. 29–30), Ron DelBene addressed the tragedy of inhibited grief among clergy and, consequently, its effect upon other people (e.g. the grandson in Smith's story and the friend in *The Big Chill*). Note these words as DelBene poignantly describes his own emotions on the death of his friend, Taylor:

> *"Taylor's death consumed me with grief ... I went through the service and out to the cemetery feeling desolate and utterly alone in my grief. At the graveside, one of my clergy friends came up and put his arms around me. 'You and Taylor were good friends, weren't you?' he said. 'Yes,' I replied. That was all it took. With my friend holding me in his arms and offering the comfort I needed, sobs came from the depths of my heart."*
>
> *Ron DelBene (1991, pp. 29–30)*

Another class of people who are expected to remain calm and stalwart are funeral directors. One funeral director explains, *"It just won't do to have the director go to pieces."* I (SLJ) performed the funeral service of a 30-year-old wife and mother of eight children; one of the children was only two days old at the time of her death. Prior to the service itself, the funeral director and I were conversing on the logistics. At one point during the dialogue, I asked him: *"Do you ever get used to this?"* He responded with, *"No, I would worry about myself if it didn't bother me."* Needless to say, that was a difficult funeral service for all involved. Lincoln Hawley (1990, p. 160), another funeral director, confirms the previous funeral director's words as well as acknowledging the emotional demands of restraint.

> *"To process the casket containing the remains of a close friend is just short of hell ... We, too, need help."*
>
> *Lincoln Hawley (1990, p. 160)*

There is one final stratum of society I want to mention in this chapter—children. Are you aware that our society inhibits children from grieving by aggressively attempting to shield them from death? Do we not frequently hear, "Oh! They are too young to understand." A logical conclusion to that statement is that children are too young to grieve. Are they? How old does a person have to be in order to grieve? Saint Francis Xavier Church's funeral planning guidebook contains these words:

> *"Children old enough to love are old enough to grieve."*
>
> *Saint Francis Xavier Church (1996)*

While it is true that a small child may not fully understand the finality of loss, he or she does realize that there has been a drastic change in the environment in which he or she lives. Pastoral care givers can be extremely helpful to families before significant damage occurs in children, especially at the funeral service.

> *"In order to avert any unintentional emotional harm to children in their grief processes, pastoral care givers should encourage adults to involve children, at least to some degree, in the memorializing and ritualizing of loved ones."*
>
> *SLJ*

This assessment is pointedly articulated in a child's words to a playmate: *"I can't come to play because I have to play with my mother."* Who said this? It was six-year-old George W. Bush, now the President of the United States, after the death of his sister, Robin (in Minutaglio, 1999).

In conclusion, Therese Rando (1984) offers these suggestions for care givers when confronted with inhibited grief:

- Review with the griever the shared relationship with the deceased. Listen for what is said and what is left unsaid. This review and your skill as a care giver may sufficiently "jump-start" the grieving.
- Communicate that you recognize the griever's inner pain and stress as well as the reluctance to grieve thoroughly and publicly. This can facilitate meaningful, healthy dialogue.
- Give permission to grieve. Be mindful that the mourner may be "inhibited" by fear or something (someone) else from releasing emotions in the presence of certain people.

- Help the griever find the right person(s) with whom he or she would feel comfortable expressing the grief.
- Many grievers are afraid that if they start to cry they will not be able to stop. They can be assured that the tears will shut themselves off after a short while.

Stacked Grief

In an ideal world, we would have only one loss to grieve at any given time. Unfortunately, grief does not check calendars for convenient scheduling. Some people are repeatedly ambushed by multiple losses; these losses can be of a simultaneous nature (e.g. automobile or plane crash) or in serial form through a relatively rapid succession of deaths, the falling domino effect. The latter can often cause the grievers to cry out "I wonder who—or what—is next?" or "Things always come in threes." In stacked grief, the bereaved do not have adequate time to grieve fully before another occasion for grief is initiated. I (HIS) had a participant in a workshop who had lost 11 family members in 18 months. Therefore, these "stackers" juggle multiple grief-causing scenarios, sometimes with others on the horizon. Among those thought more susceptible to the possibility of "stacked grief" are:

- senior adults whose family/social network is shrinking
- survivors of disasters
- individuals in dangerous, "high risk" occupations (police, fire, emergency service providers, etc.)
- military personnel in combat theaters
- healthcare professionals, particularly in nursing homes and hospices
- individuals experiencing a succession of deaths in family/social circles
- individuals balancing losses through death with significant losses of another kind.

Stacked grief is particularly troublesome for elderly adults as their families and social networks slowly or rapidly disappear. This is especially true when some of the deceased were those special family members or friends to whom the griever would have turned for support. I (HIS) remember my mother's lament.

"A whole lot of people are leaving here."

HIS

I did not fully understand what she meant by that statement until I addressed her Christmas cards one year. Name after name after name had been crossed out in her address book—deceased. Similar to the words of Mrs. Smith were those of my father upon a return from a high-school class reunion:

"The crowd keeps getting smaller year after year."

HIS

One senior adult chided friends at another funeral with dark humor, "We've got to stop meeting like this." Pastoral care givers can provide an invaluable service for the elderly bereaved in helping them to identify support systems. Joy Johnson relates a story about Lord Snowdon who made a film about elderly British royalty. He asked one duke what was the most difficult thing about growing old. The very proper gentleman replied, "The deaths of one's contemporaries, definitely." (Personal correspondence, 2006).

Stacked grief can be acute for survivors of disasters as well as family and friends of victims/survivors. Think of fire officers and police in New York who lost several friends and colleagues in the World Trade Center or Pentagon attacks. Survivors often feel very blessed and jubilant to be "alive," while at the same time, there are feelings of survivor guilt for "being alive" in the midst of massive grief. "Why did I survive? I am no more special than all the others who died." This latter feeling is coincident with the grief they are experiencing. The other side of that, however, is the wish to die to end the suffering associated with the guilt of survival. Primarily, though, it is victims' loved ones who experience stacked grief in its fullest sense.

Ponder the case concerning teen-aged students of Mortonsville, Pennsylvania. Sixteen students in the city's high school French Club, en route for a summer study experience in Paris, France, were killed in the July 17, 1996 crash of TWA Flight 800. The result of that horrific tragedy was stacked grief especially because of the media fascination. Set aside for a moment the devastating blow that it was to family members and consider the impact upon the students' friends, even the citizens of that community. Dealing with the loss of one friend is demanding, but multiplied many times over, it can become unbearable.

> *"Care givers can create an oasis in the lonely desert of death."*
>
> *SLJ*

Individuals in dangerous occupations are not immune to stacked grief, even though they are fully aware that serious injury and death go along with the territory of the profession. Law enforcement officers, firefighters, emergency service person-nel, and military service personnel are members of some of the more obvious professions wherein danger is an ever-present companion. In line-of-duty deaths in multiple increments of one or in mass, stacked grief permeates not only depart-ments, but large sectors of the profession. Law enforcement officers from far and wide assemble for honoring fallen comrades; the same is true for the heroic dead in firefighters' ranks. Unfortunately, guilt can also be an unwelcome bedfellow in line-of-duty deaths.

> *"If somebody had to die in that fire, it should have been me, not him. He had a wife and three small children."*

> *"She shouldn't have died in that exchange of gunfire. She had her whole life ahead of her. She was engaged, about to be married; she was so happy."*

A domino-like succession of deaths can happen within a given family just as it can happen in a particular high-risk vocation. This may happen to adult children when an elderly mother dies and two months later their father, or stepfather, dies when they find themselves simultaneously mourning both parents.

In August 1989, my (SLJ) wife's paternal grandfather died on a Sunday; the following Sunday, my maternal grandfather died. I performed two funerals in one week for family members. In February 1993, my wife's paternal grandmother died; two days later, my paternal grandmother died; the next day, my paternal grand-father died. This time, I conducted three funerals for family members in one week. Now, I realize that these scenarios are rare. Nevertheless, it is not uncommon for elderly uncles, aunts, parents, grandparents to die in close proximity of one another and, thereby, begin something of a chain reaction within families. In such cases, a little paranoia might come into the picture: "Well, who will the *next one* be? When will it happen again?" Every ring of the telephone is dreaded.

Multiple deaths in one occurrence or the same resulting from an accumulation of numerous events are not the only occasions for stacked grief. In fact, stacked grief can happen with non-death losses, it can happen through a series of multiple significant losses at one time or a series of losses over time. For example, an individual can lose his job of 20 years through downsizing, and his wife can lose her health to the degree that she has to have constant care. Both of these result in the loss of the dreamed retirement. Does this qualify those involved to be experiencing stacked grief? It absolutely does. Senior adults, because of the death of a spouse or care giver, may experience the loss of a home (move in with adult children, nursing home, assisted-living facility), a garden, precious memories, neighborhood, independence through driving, daily interactions with friends and neighbors, etc. The role of the deceased as a support person for the bereaved often leaves the bereaved feeling lost—no one to turn to; does not know where to go or what to do.

Stacked grief has been compared to riding bumper cars. Once you recover from one hit, **BAM!**, you get hit again. Stacked grief is a reality of increasing proportions in our society as it becomes more violent, older, and more seriously diseased. To administer adequate pastoral care in situations of stacked grief, we recommend the following suggestions.

- Stacked grief survivors may be dealing with "bereavement overload," a term coined by Robert J. Kastenbaum in an article entitled "Death and Bereavement in Later Life" (1969). This was especially true of gay men who lost large friend networks early in the AIDS epidemic or youths who have lost multiple friends in accidents, suicides, acts of violence. Legal proceedings and media coverage may further contribute to the feeling of "overload."
- Moreover, those who would normally have supported the grievers may be among the deceased. In order for a person to deal with the latest loss, a pastoral care giver may have to help the griever "audit," process, or prioritize all of the losses.
- In some cases, it will be impossible to deal with all the losses. This is especially true in situations of massive, multiple losses in one occurrence. Therefore, the pastoral care giver may want to focus on the latest loss or a particular loss. Then, determine some ways that the griever can deal intentionally and deliberately with or symbolize that loss.

This discussion might have given the impression that people experiencing stacked grief may have difficulty dealing with the losses for long periods of time. That may be true for some people but not for others. This same concept holds true for people experiencing grief of any type. Jane Brody cited some findings from the "Report on Bereavement and Grief" conducted by the Center for Advancement of Health in the February 1, 2004 edition of the *New York Times* (Brody, 2004):

- Most people do not experience "problematic" grief or have adverse health effects.
- Some people do not experience distress after being bereaved.
- Positive emotions are possible after a loss.

Doka contends as well that people in general do not need as much time to resolve a loss. A reason for this may well be that people are receiving more support and grieve their losses in more healthy ways.

> *"I hope you can find the healing power in grieving."*
> Morrie Schwartz in Tuesdays with Morrie (Albom, 1997, p. 86)

Traumatic Grief

September 11, 2001 will be forever etched into the minds of Americans of all ages. People will remember where they were and what they were doing when those four jets crashed into New York City's World Trade Center, the Pentagon in Washington, DC and the remote area of western Pennsylvania. Likewise, July 7, 2005 will be remembered by the people of Great Britain. They will remember where they were when those bombs exploded on the public transit system in London. The grief resulting from that violent act of terrorism is little short of debilitating for multiplied thousands of people.

In April 1991, United States Attorney General, Janet Reno, reported that *"A citizen of this country is more likely to be a victim of a violent crime than of an automobile accident."* Furthermore, Thomas Radecki, Research Director for the National Coalition on Television Violence, suggested that by age 18 the average American child will have seen 200,000 violent acts on television, which includes 40,000 murders. Moreover, real-life violence and death of a traumatic nature have become common television news. Given the globalization of society, especially Western society, tragedies in the remotest part of the world become part of our "daily mix of news."

> *"Violence contributes significantly to the increasing prevalence of complicated mourning."*
> Therese Rando (1992–93, p. 48)

How true Rando's words are. Not only is it the violent nature of the act itself which complicates mourning, but the public attention such receives. Violence and death become lead stories in the around-the-clock news, and no angle of the story is too small to analyze or, as some families would argue, over-analyze. Thus, families and friends must grieve in the glare of public scrutiny and fascination, unable to grieve in private. Furthermore, this public interest can be of a lengthy duration, lasting through criminal and/or civil litigation.

According to Drs. Jeffrey T. Mitchell and George S. Everly, founders of the International Critical Incident Stress Foundation (ICISF), excessive media interest qualifies something resulting in a significant loss to be designated as a *critical incident*, which they define as *"any event which has enough emotional power to overwhelm a person's (or group's) ability to cope"* (Mitchell and Everly, 1997). The result of that horrific event may well be the onset of post traumatic stress (PTS), which Mitchell defines as *"a normal reaction in a normal person to an abnormal event."* It is important to note, though, that "any" death has the potential to be a critical incident in the eyes of the bereaved. Unless people with PTS receive adequate care, they can develop post traumatic stress disorder (PTSD). PTSD might also be termed "traumatic grief."

However, it is not only intentional, violent acts against others that produce PTS, PTSD, and traumatic grief. Mitchell cites a number of things that qualify as well:

- suicide
- serious life-threatening event to self
- prolonged incident, especially one which ends in a loss
- events involving children
- disasters/multi-casualty incidents
- killing or wounding someone by accident.

Consider the Valujet plane crash in the Florida Everglades when family members were flown to a location near the crash site where they waited for the recovery of loved ones' bodies, or body parts in some instances. Under normal circumstances, the Everglades is a beautiful, peaceful place, alive with all kinds of creatures, most notably large alligators. In this instance, the sight of the murky waters and alligators added immeasurable anxiety to the victim's families. "Will my loved one ever be found? Was her body eaten by an alligator?" These people experienced a critical incident event causing PTS, resulting in, for many, PTSD and traumatic grief. However, people do not have to witness events or visit places to have PTS or develop PTSD; experiencing vicariously can also be the catalyst for the stress-related disorder.

> *"Accidents also throw us off balance. They catch us off guard and force us to live with anxiety and the unknown. We sense we can no longer provide safety for ourselves or someone dear to us. This sense of losing control can be traumatizing."*
>
> *Dan Bagby (1999, p. 96)*

Traumatic grief is closely related to destructive and stacked grief. In fact, it may be fair to say that unchecked destructive and stacked grief becomes traumatic grief, which is becoming more prevalent. We live in a culture where *an act of violence occurs every two seconds*. Because of this, pastoral care is commonly dispensed in that culture of trauma and violence. Therefore, pastoral issues for consideration are many.

- As a pastoral care giver, you may be asked for your opinion on viewing the body, no viewing, or limited viewing. Consultation with the funeral director prior to offering your counsel is prudent. One additional point to keep in mind, before you offer your suggestion, is that lack of viewing may interfere with the acceptance of death (Alan Wolfelt, *Creating Meaningful Funeral Rituals: A Guide for Care Givers*, 1994). And individuals may imagine the body looking far worse; thus, for some, viewing can reduce the trauma.
- As a memorial service leader, you may be asked to make concessions to accommodate a more public funeral and burial, thereby making allowances for media coverage. Unless pastoral care givers offer firm leadership and are sensitive to the family, a funeral can be "hijacked" and turned into a media circus.
- In disasters or other situations of a traumatic nature, pastoral care givers often attract the interest of the media looking for a certain "twist" on the hot story. In these situations, it is quite possible to make innocent blunders that compromise confidentiality or say things that may be misinterpreted by family as well as community and faith congregation members. Kelly Smith offers some advice for

care givers in an article entitled "Ten Tips for Tough Times" (1999, p. 32); some of those tips are:
  - make sure you have authority to speak to the press
  - if you are uncomfortable doing an interview, do not do it
  - avoid immediate "on the spot" live interviews
  - anything you say may be used against you or against … your faith congregation/organization
  - "no comment" may be interpreted that you are hiding something
  - ask yourself: "How will the family 'see' this interview?"
- In cases of disaster, pastoral care givers, who are often considered as God's representatives, may be asked to comment on a variety of assumptions about God, now under scrutiny because of the sadness and severity of the tragedy. "How could a God of love cause this?" "If there is a God in heaven …" "Where is hope in all of this?" Remember this: God does not need to be defended. Acknowledge the feelings and relate that it is okay to question and even be angry at God. Also, gently and in the appropriate time, assure the bereaving that God has not abandoned them. On the contrary, God is with them in the midst of the trauma.
- In situations of traumatic grief, a major goal is stabilization (a primary goal in crisis intervention) to prevent escalating distress. The resultant goal is to bring about a restoration of balance and the ability to adapt and function. It is also important to enable people to start talking about the event as soon as possible, albeit without being forceful.

Mitchell and Everly developed a program called Critical Incident Stress Management (CISM). During the training sessions, they point out that critical incidents may cause physical, cognitive, emotional, behavioral, and spiritual reactions which can overwhelm anyone's usual abilities to cope. These are normal responses that can last a few days, a few weeks, a few months, and occasionally longer depending upon the severity of the traumatic experience. Interestingly, in some cases, weeks or months may pass before any stress reactions manifest themselves. One important consideration is that these responses do not imply weakness, only that the particular incident was too much for a person(s) to manage alone, and they are resolvable. As pastoral care givers, you should be aware of some of the common reactions shown in Box 3.2.

Use caution when attempting to conduct critical incident stress management techniques (e.g. defusing, debriefing) without training. Furthermore, the issues in traumatic grief are often of the magnitude that the care givers themselves may well need care given to them as well. Thus, it would be advisable for any care giver to have a group of care givers available as needed. Since whole person care involves addressing concerns of the body, mind, and spirit, the care giver's resource group would ideally include a medical professional, a mental health professional and a clergy person.

Box 3.2   Some Common Stress Reactions

Physical Reactions

Fatigue	Rapid heart rate
Nausea	Thirst
Dizziness	Grinding of teeth
Headaches	Weakness
Sleep disturbances	Chills
Muscle tremors	Fainting
Profuse sweating	Twitches
Digestive problems	Elevated blood pressure

Cognitive Reactions

Difficulty concentrating	Difficulty solving problems
Difficulty making decisions	Poor problem solving
Difficulty in performing familiar tasks	Difficulty in naming familiar things
Heightened or lowered alertness	Preoccupation with the incident
Flashbacks of the incident	Difficulty in remembering
Nightmares	Poor abstract thinking
Need to blame someone	Disturbed thinking

Emotional Reactions

Fear	*Irritability*
Guilt	*Emotional numbing*
Depression	*Identification with the victim*
Anxiety	*Uncertainty*
Apprehension	*Agitation*
Intense anger	*Feeling overwhelmed*
Emotional shock	*Denial*

Behavioral Reactions

Change in activity	Change in speech patterns
Withdrawal	Alcohol consumption
Inability to rest	Antisocial acts
Change in sexual functioning	Erratic movements
Startle reflex intensified	Hyper-alertness to environment
Loss or increase of appetite	Pacing
Emotional outbursts	Hyper/sluggish activity

Spiritual Reactions

Sense of hopelessness	Sudden turn toward God
Anger at God	Belief that God is powerless
"God's will" mindset	Loss of meaning and purpose
"Why me?" syndrome	Belief that God does not care
Feeling distant from God	Belief that "I failed God"
Sense of isolation from God and faith community	Questioning of basic beliefs of one's faith
Familiar faith practices seem empty	Uncharacteristic congregational involvement
Withdrawal from faith congregation	Belief that God is not in control

"The loss of human lives, especially children, is inherently overwhelming."
Jeffrey T. Mitchell (1999)

Mitchell's words were in reference to the loss of lives due to a critical incident. However, his words can also be understood in the most general of senses—the loss of anyone dear to you in any manner is overwhelming. There are three books, among many, that we would highly recommend for ministry with those experiencing traumatic grief:

- *The Minister as Crisis Counselor* by David Switzer (1974)
- *Critical Incident Stress Management* by George S. Everly and Jeffrey T. Mitchell (1999)
- *Critical Incident Stress Debriefing: An Operations Manual* by Jeffrey T. Mitchell and George S. Everly (1997).

We conclude this chapter with these words by Jeffrey T. Mitchell ("We Remember!" *Life Net*, **10**(4), a publication of the International Critical Incident Stress Foundation, Inc.):

"You do not honor the memory ... by losing faith, or obsessively contemplating ... sinking into pathological grief or into the depths of despair ... You honor the memory of these special people by drawing closer to those you love now and by appreciating the beauty of their lives. You honor their memory by taking on life in its fullest ... laugh and to feel joy and to appreciate a flower, enjoy the view from a mountain, play a game, have a party ..."
Jeffrey T. Mitchell (1999)

4

When a Baby Dies: The Loss of a Dream

Death is a human experience that confronts all of us with our own mortality. This is especially true when the object of death is someone our own age or slightly younger. However, one of the most overwhelming and devastating experiences with death for any family, particularly parents, is the death of a child. Note these words of Al Miles:

> *"Whether the child dies during the first trimester of pregnancy, at or shortly after birth, from an accident or terminal disease, in home, hospital, or hospice, as an adolescent, or in adulthood, parents and family members are devastated by this tragedy. The natural order of life has been disrupted."*
>
> *Al Miles (1995, p. 40)*

"The natural order of life has been disrupted." That is so very true when people die whose parents or grandparents are still alive. Children are supposed to bury their parents, not vice versa. Furthermore, the pain and suffering associated with a child's death cannot be measured. The June 13, 2002 issue of *The Wall Street Journal* featured an article entitled "In the Words of Parents Who Lost Kids." In the editorial, the author quoted from one of the stories of more than 250 bereaved parents:

> *"If people could visually see our wounds, they'd see we've been opened from neck to pelvis, with all our insides hanging out."*
>
> *Wall Street Journal (June 13, 2002)*

In situations such as these, the justness of life (or, in reality, death) becomes an issue with which the survivors often grapple. When a death appears to be quite unjust, the justness of God is also a concern which grievers may address. According to Gary Vogel in *A Caregiver's Handbook to Perinatal Loss* (1996, p. 59), there is probably no more unjust death than that of an innocent child.

> *"Parents never expect to outlive their children, even the unborn."*
>
> *SLJ*

In this chapter, we turn our attention to the grief associated with perinatal loss, which includes the following:

- ectopic pregnancy (tubal pregnancy)
- miscarriage (varies in designation among states: e.g. in Kansas, it refers to weight, less than 350 grams–11 ounces; in many states, miscarriage refers to gestation less than 20 weeks)

- stillbirth (varies in designation among states: e.g. in Kansas, it refers to weight, more than 350 grams–11 ounces; in many states, stillbirth refers to gestation more than 20 weeks)
- neonatal (infant) death.

According to Kellner and Lake (1990) and Rando (1986), whenever perinatal loss occurs, other losses also occur.

- Parents lose their dreams and hopes for the child.
- Parents lose a part of themselves.
- Parents lose a part of each other.
- Parents lose their future, especially if the perinatal loss results in the inability to have children.

However, the field of losses should be expanded because other people experience and grieve the loss:

- siblings
- grandparents, who experience dual losses:
  1. loss of their grandchild
  2. loss in feelings of helplessness concerning their child who is hurting so badly (this is discussed later in this chapter)
- family friends
- hospital personnel, especially nurses.

Unfortunately, while that broad, expansive field of grievers is understood with other losses, it is less evident in perinatal loss. Why is that? Unfortunately, to the general public, which includes many pastoral care givers, the loss was not "really" a loss. According to Miles:

> *"Many people assume that since the baby never lived outside the mother's womb and only a few weeks in utero, that the grief parents experience is far less traumatic than the grief experienced by parents who suffer the death of an older child."*
>
> *Al Miles (1995, p. 37).*

With that in mind, ponder these words of Rick Wheat:

> *"Grieving over a miscarriage is uniquely difficult because it is so unlike any other loss. Miscarriage takes much more than a couple's expected future baby. Dreams are shattered. A future pregnancy with the delightful possibilities of parenthood is stolen. Both partners hold the empty knowledge that the people they might have been, if only their child had been born, will not be."*
>
> *Rick Wheat (1996, p. 32)*

Some mothers actually experience some symptoms of post traumatic stress (e.g. intrusive thoughts). Most parents who have experienced perinatal loss would welcome the opportunity of talking about their losses, dreams, and aspirations. However, no one invites them to do so. That statement is validated by the story of a Pennsylvania woman who gave birth to a stillborn baby girl and displays her daughter's footprints in a frame on her desk at work. The mother regretfully said: "Only one person has commented on it" (*The Wall Street Journal*, June 13, 2002).

Thus, perinatal grievers experience abandonment, which is extremely lonely in nature, in two forms:

1. initial—in the first hours, days, weeks after the loss; no meal brought to the home, no flowers, no obituary in the local newspaper, no ritual
2. long-term—no mention of the loss in conversations as would be the case with other deaths.

From whom do perinatal grievers experience abandonment?

- Spouse/parent of the child.
- Grandparents/great-grandparents and other family members.
- Healthcare professionals.
- Friends.
- Faith community.

This grief is compounded by some common perceptions concerning perinatal loss.

- Perinatal grievers were expected to grieve quickly, quietly, and alone.
- There were few rituals for perinatal loss.
- Perinatal loss was believed to be less significant than other losses, even that of a pet.
- Children were cremated and often unnamed.
- Parents were often advised to have another baby as soon as possible to "replace" the deceased child.

Furthermore, when grief for perinatal loss is recognized and affirmed, the attention is generally focused upon the mother. This is especially true in a hospital setting where "she" is the patient. How, then, does this apparent neglect of attention appear to the baby's father? Note these words of Brett O'Neill, a grieving father:

> *"I found it very difficult when people would ask how my wife was and ignore my needs. Perhaps this is the double-edged sword of being strong on the outside and being expected to cope, but crying out on the inside for someone to ask how I was."*
> *Brett O'Neill (1998, p. 35)*

Why is an inordinate amount of attention given to one of the parents (mother) to the exclusion of the other (father)? There are a variety of reasons for this.

- There is the common belief that mothers express higher levels of grief and grieve longer than the fathers because mothers' grief is shaped by the physiological attachment to the child:
  - carrying the baby in her womb
  - physical restrictions during pregnancy
  - complications from the death
  - constant reminder of the child because of the lingering presence of breast milk.

  > *"No one knows what it is like to carry your purse in your lap rather than your baby when you leave the hospital."*
  > *Mother of two stillborn babies*

- Given the number of women electing to have a baby without commitment in a relationship, the father may be excluded by the mother of any involvement in her life or that of the baby.

- The father is expected to keep a "level head," assume more responsibility for the household and, in general, "be strong" for the mother who has been physically and emotionally traumatized.

Women tend to become attached to the baby once the pregnancy is known and dream of the pregnancy, infancy, early life of the baby. Men, on the other hand, tend to imagine the child at an older age—playing sports, fun in the park, etc. This is not to say, though, that men have no attachment to the baby during pregnancy. The father's attachment to the unborn is, generally speaking, simply less in the early stages of the pregnancy than in the latter stages. Because of this, a father's grief may be less intense and shorter in duration in miscarriages early in pregnancy than those further on in the process or a stillbirth. Nevertheless, a father still grieves, even though it may be hidden from public view. Tears in a male often equal sobbing in a female.

There are other losses that parents encounter in addition to the loss of their baby: financial and domestic. With respect to financial loss, a family economic crisis can ensue because of the pregnancy. In some pregnancies of a problematic nature, working mothers have had to quit work and stay home, sometimes in bed for weeks or even be hospitalized. In cases where pregnancies were unplanned or there is no insurance coverage, even a normal pregnancy can severely hamper a family's financial situation when they are totally responsible for the costs associated with the pregnancy. That is not to mention how financially devastating a problem-laden pregnancy can be. Of course, the problem of finances is added to the loss of the child. The combination of the two can also lead to problems in the marriage, thus compounding the grief.

Sexual intimacy can be impacted by perinatal loss. Wallerstedt and Higgins (1996) report that fathers tend to desire sexual relations before mothers:

> *"Fathers tend to view sexual activity as comforting and sharing, and reasonable (particularly if they had been abstinent during late pregnancy) but often the mothers, because their grief was so intense, perceived the father to be uncaring, unsensitized."*
>
> *Wallerstedt and Higgins (1996, p. 391)*

In reality, many men consider having sex as an expression of tenderness. One mother told a grief group: "I just couldn't believe it when he made his move on me. And then he proceeded to try to talk me into it. I was totally put off and went to sleep in the guest room." When emotions are high, as in times like the loss of a baby, it is easy to understand how a grieving mother could feel "put upon" by her husband or partner. It is equally easy to understand how a father might feel hurt or even angered when rejected.

The reverse of this scenario is also true. The father can feel that sexual intimacy is inappropriate. Immediately following a baby's death, a mother may experience an intense urge to become pregnant again. It is a natural tendency to attempt desperately to find that precious something one has lost. The father, on the other hand, may be resistant, recalling that it was the sexual act itself which was the catalyst for the present experience—a dead baby. The result of the father's rejection of the mother's romantic overtures can hurt or anger her. This rejection can also induce guilt feelings in the mother: "You think it was my fault our baby died?"

Therese Rando argues that the disinterest in sex is mutual among grieving parents. She suggests that they may feel guilty experiencing the pleasure of sexual intimacy while grieving. She goes on to say that relations can be *"compromised by disinterest, depression or avoidance as long as two years"* (1986, p. 29). This is particularly the case for couples with previous relational, financial, or communication difficulties.

Perinatal loss not only affects sexual intimacy but the relationship as a whole. Because of the complex difficulties of perinatal loss, there is a common belief that it leads to divorce, or at least separation, at rates as high as 80% plus. Recent data, though, challenges those ratings as mere exaggerations. In fact, a study conducted by The Compassionate Friends concluded that only 12% of couples suffering perinatal loss divorced (NFO Research, 1999, p. 11). One wonders if that percentage would have been substantially lower had there been adequate pastoral care following the loss.

Certainly, for some, the death of a child can be the proverbial "straw that broke the camel's back" in already strained relationships. In some cases, the death of the baby provides at least one party in the relationship the motivation to terminate the relationship before another pregnancy. On the other hand, a reason for an immediate attempt at another pregnancy is to "keep us together."

However, interesting studies by Page-Liberman and Hughes (1990) and Kimble (1991) place a different twist on these perceptions. Their studies found that more than half of the fathers surveyed reported that they had grown closer to the mothers as a result of the loss. One father explained that the new closeness came as result of *"having gone through hell together"* (Kimble, 1991, p. 48). Furthermore, according to Menke and McClead (1990), grief forces re-examinations of and reflections upon the relationship, which bring the grieving couple closer.

Without question, perinatal loss can significantly strain even the strongest of relationships. The astute pastoral care giver should be careful to observe any warning signals of relational distress following perinatal loss. A 1998 publication by Bereavement Services entitled *It Means So Much To Know That Someone Cares* has identified several warning signals worthy of consideration:

- spending more time at work
- an extramarital affair
- an increase in the use of alcohol or other recreational drugs
- over-involvement in one's faith community or other groups
- over-protectiveness of a surviving child or children
- spending an inordinate amount of time with parents, siblings, friends
- prolonged lack of sexual activity
- lack of communication (i.e. sharing of feelings).

With respect to the last warning signal, note the four factors cited by Kennell, Slyter, and Klaus (1970) which influence successful, healthy grief, both positively and negatively:

1. poor communication between parents
2. previous losses
3. positive feelings about the pregnancy (i.e. was it wanted by both?)
4. having touched or held the baby before burial or death if delivered alive.

It is certain that, among the other factors mentioned, communication between parents will be challenged by perinatal loss. Because of the detriment caused in relationships due to poor communication, the goal is to enhance communication with the hope of achieving that which is described by Wallerstedt and Higgins (1996):

> *"Bereaved parents often experience an intense level of personal growth and maturity that allows them to develop more effective communication skills, which strengthen their relationship."*
>
> *Wallerstedt and Higgins (1996, p. 391)*

Effective pastoral care with perinatal loss grievers can help to facilitate that growth which will enhance the couple's relationship. It is to that subject we now turn our attention.

Pastoral Care and Perinatal Loss

What parents really want is for family, friends and loved ones to acknowledge their loss.

> *"People never said dead, death or loss to us. I wanted to hear these words because then at least I felt they had some sense of our great loss and pain."*
>
> *The Wall Street Journal, June 13, 2002*

These words were expressed by a young mother whose baby was not alive when delivered. She went on to say that she and her husband received the greatest support in their grief from their other children and the hospital chaplain, not family, friends, or faith community. Is the case of Doug and Kate an isolated one? Unfortunately, it is not.

Remember Kate's words: People never said *dead, death, loss*. And yet, that is what happened. Amanda (the baby's name) died; she was dead. That is the one message that the community in general and pastoral care givers in particular need to hear: Perinatal loss is a death which devastates many parents. Why is it then that the many parents who experience such losses are not vocal about them? It might well be because such losses are not deemed by society as what they really are: the death of a human being. Thus, public grief over something "minor" is a social taboo.

Unfortunately, few people are aware that mothers who miscarry early in pregnancy may experience the same intensity of grief as those who carry the baby full-term resulting in a stillbirth. Eileen Connell, Perinatal Bereavement Coordinator of Shawnee Mission Medical Center, Shawnee Mission, Kansas, states: *"Studies suggest that 75–80 percent of mothers who miscarry view the experience as the loss of a child."* Connell goes on to say that the appropriate response to such losses is two-fold:

1. they need to be recognized
2. they need to be validated.

One way to recognize and validate the loss is to encourage naming the baby and using that name when talking with the family. The rest of this chapter will address other ways to recognize and validate perinatal losses.

According to Gary Vogel, the most haunting question grieving parents ask is "Why?" This question is most often addressed in the context of one's religious belief system. However, since most people believe that their belief systems are fair (God or the gods are benevolent), the "why" question will shift to "why us?" (Vogel, 1996, p. 60):

- "What did we do to deserve this?"
- "Why did this pregnancy fail?"
- "We are good people, why did this have to happen to us?"
- "Why, God?"

Vogel continues that this questioning of God is usually done in anger, which is itself a key element in grief. For many people, this anger at God is followed by guilt for their anger at God. The guilt already felt for the death of the child is compounded by guilt for being angry at God. What these grieving parents need to know is that it is understandable they are angry at God, and it is okay to be so. Grieving families need to hear repeatedly:

> "It is okay to be angry, even angry at God. At whom do we vent anxieties, frustrations, anger? Is it not the people who love and care for us? Why do we choose them? Because we know they will not reject us. No one loves us more than God. He will not reject us for being angry at Him for He understands our pain. In fact, He will draw us ever closer to Himself when He knows we are hurting."
>
> SLJ

Grieving parents need to be affirmed that their questions and feelings of anger, despair, and frustration are normal and acceptable.

Harold Ivan Smith relates that the most important gift pastoral care givers can bring to those in perinatal grief is to hurt with them. Care givers also must admit that they cannot take away this hurt with anything they might say. Audit the family: who might need a compassionate word from me? The death of a baby might be hard on the first-time grandfather or grandmother. In fact, Gary Vogel suggests that *"erasing the pain is not something to be aspired to anyway, in that, at the moment the pain may be all the parents feel they have left to honor their baby"* (1996, p. 62). Listening in silence is a major key in providing support to perinatal grieving parents (Miles, 1995, p. 37). A pastoral care giver cannot give an answer for why the loss occurred except to say that we live in a world where bad things happen, even to good people.

Furthermore, one cannot say, "I know how you feel," even if that person has experienced a similar loss, for each death and the grief associated with it are unique (Limbo *et al.*, 1986, p. 127). The best gift a pastoral care giver or anyone can give grievers is to listen and to listen some more:

- "I am willing to talk about it with you."
- "I am willing to cry with you."
- "I am willing to hurt with you."
- "I am willing to listen to you."

Simply being there is often the best offer of support for the grief-stricken.

Moreover, one thing that should *never* be said when a baby dies, or anyone for that matter, is, "It is God's will." William Sloane Coffin, Jr. said that *"God is against all unnatural deaths,"* and what can be a death more unnatural than that of a baby: born or unborn. *"There is no fairness to such a loss. However, if families see that God is with them in their sorrow, they may find comfort in the midst of the tragedy"* (Limbo *et al.*, 1986, p. 126). Pastoral care givers can communicate God's presence with the bereaved as representatives, not to answer for or defend God. In fact, even "God language" is not altogether necessary, and platitudes, most assuredly, should be avoided at all times. The first of many to avoid has already been mentioned: "It is God's will." Miles and Vogel suggest a number of others to avoid (Miles, 1995, p. 38; Vogel, 1996, p. 62):

- "You now have a little angel in heaven."
- "You are young, so you can have other children."
- "Thank God, you have other children."
- "Your child is better off now."
- "You seem to be handling this so well."
- "This experience will make you stronger."
- "This is for the best."
- "I know how you feel."
- "It could have been a lot worse."
- "We know that in everything God works for good."
- "We shouldn't grieve as others who have no hope."
- "God is taking care of your baby now."

Some of these have been referred to previously, and others will be discussed subsequently when we address pastoral issues. You, of course, notice the references to God in these clichés, which are supposed to comfort grieving people. However, as opposed to providing comfort, to many, they are just hollow words—words that incite contempt, anger, indifference.

Any reference to God in an attempt to comfort the bereaved of perinatal loss should be tempered with a message similar to this from William Sloane Coffin, Jr.:

> *"... when the waves closed over the sinking car, God's heart was the first of all our hearts to break."*
>
> *William Sloane Coffin, Jr.*

Now, concerning issues for pastoral care givers to perinatal grievers, Burke and Matsumoto identify multiple roles that a chaplain can fill in support of medical and support staff in perinatal and neonatal environments (1999). These roles can also fulfill some of the needs of grieving parents:

- creator of meaning
- trustworthy listener
- calming presence
- pastoral presence
- fellow sojourner in the land of bereavement
- grief educator to encourage such things as bathing, powdering, holding, naming, etc.
- generator of ethical concerns.

We will now list and discuss other issues of concern for pastoral care givers of perinatal loss grievers.

- **Make clear that perinatal loss is not unlike grief resulting from any other death.** Because of this fact, there should be no attempts to make the family feel better (which in reality only succeeds in minimizing the loss) by the use of evasive, placating statements. However, there is one sense in which perinatal loss is unique. The grief associated with perinatal death can continually resurface if the couple has or will have other children by the asking of a common question: "How many children do you have?" Some couples do not know how to respond: "Do I count the deceased baby?" "If I do, will that complicate or terminate the conversation?"

- **Grant the parents permission to do thorough grief.** As a pastoral care giver, you must remember that this is a significant loss. One word of caution, though: do not attempt to put more "grief" on the couple than exists. Quite honestly, for some parents, a miscarriage is not as significant a loss as it is for others. Sensitivity is the key in assessing the situation. There are many ways to grant permission. Perhaps the best way is to be there and encourage them that it is okay to hurt. However, one needs to be careful how this counsel is communicated. Nancy Crump relates hearing these words from a grieving mother.

> *"I don't need your permission to hurt."*
>
> *A grieving mother*

- **Caution against having another child "as soon as possible" for *this* loss must be recognized and grieved.** Perinatal grievers often have an intense desire to get pregnant again in order to "replace" the lost baby. Through the passage of time, this frantic urge diminishes, thus providing the opportunity for rational contemplation of a future pregnancy. It is in the later time of reflection that grieving parents come to realize that having another child will not replace the one who died.

- Furthermore, the birth of any subsequent child brings with it the potential for crisis in the realization that "this" baby did not replace the miscarried or stillborn child. Therefore, this couple may experience mixed feelings of grief and joy simultaneously. Moreover, future pregnancies will most likely be more anxiety-laden. The innocence of and immunity from problematic births is long gone. In most cases, a sufficient lapse of time between the loss and a future pregnancy is advisable. Conversely, counsel to consider an immediate subsequent pregnancy is revolting to many young couples. Note these words of a grieving young mother.

> *"When Doug told the doctor I was 35, the doctor said, 'That's good, she will be able to have others.' I will never forget those words. They made me want to scream to the doctor, 'I don't want any others, I want this baby.'"*
>
> *Miles (1995, p. 36)*

- **Remember that grief will be activated by the holidays and other special days.** A first Mother's Day and Father's Day can be extremely difficult, as well as religious holidays which are intended to be joyous occasions for celebration. Harold Ivan Smith states that he will long remember an incident which happened in a grief group coinciding with the Christmas season. He relates that a woman participant reached into her purse, pulled out a Hallmark "Baby's First Christmas" ornament, turned to him, and demanded: "Well, Mr. Grief Expert, what am I supposed to do with this now?" Out of the midst of silence following that outburst of emotion, a grieving father participating in the group spoke up: "You hang it on the tree. That's what we did with ours. My baby is having a first Christmas in heaven."

- Hannah Lothrop in *Help, Comfort and Hope After Losing Your Baby in Pregnancy or the First Year* suggests that parents need more support during the second half of the bereavement year and into the next year because *"they are searching more deeply for meaning and a new spiritual context"* (p. 209). Miles (1995) urges pastoral care givers to write notes and encourages others to remember bereaved parents on the following dates:
  - child's birth date or due date
  - child's due date (if a premature infant)
  - anniversary of the death
  - special holidays.
- Additionally there are those "life-long dates" that challenge grievers emotionally:
  - first day of school
  - graduation
  - career
  - marriage
  - children.
- **Hear out the grief of everyone touched by the death.** Give individuals sufficient time to find words for the death. In many cases, you will be talking to the parents. Indeed, neither of them may have found a safe place to give grief its voice. Reflecting upon his own experience with perinatal loss, O'Neill expresses a concern for the necessity of healthcare and pastoral care professionals to have more interest in the needs of the grieving father. He writes: *"My grief, while being expressed intermittently, was not a priority"* (1998, p. 33). "Everyone" includes fathers, children, and grandparents. One grandmother's words were cited in Bereavement Services (1998):

  "We hurt twice. We hurt for our children because they are our children. Plus, we hurt for the grandchild we lost."

  Bereavement Services (1998)

- This group of grievers also includes healthcare professionals involved in patient care of the bereaved family. Nobody ever gets used to death, especially those which are so untimely.

  "Hearing a story is different than a medical history, for a story is as deeply imbedded in a life as cancer cells are in the body."

  SLJ

- **Be alert to related or collateral issues which compound grief.** One of these issues may be finance. Sometimes, parents may radically curtail spending in order for the mother to stop working and pay close attention to having a healthy pregnancy, and then the unthinkable happens. Contrast this with the fact that other people they knew did none of that and had healthy births and babies. The "why" question is quite understandable in such instances. Another issue could be a previous abortion—an abortion of which the father may be unaware. Imagine the questions which surface: "Was it my fault?" "Was it something related to my abortion that caused my baby to be born dead?" Somewhat related to that is a previous perinatal loss. One bereaved father relates his feelings in Bereavement Services (1998):

  "With the first pregnancy, there was so much joy and excitement, with the second one, we were afraid to get too excited."

  Bereavement Services (1998)

- Finally, parents may have to deal with the death of a twin or others from triplets, etc. and the survival of the others. Thus, they are forced to confront *"conflicting emotions of mourning the dead baby and become increasingly attached to the living one"* (Cuisinier *et al.*, 1996, p. 339). In such instances, one shudders when some well-meaning people say: "Think about what you have rather than what you have lost." Pastoral care givers can help in such situations by encouraging grief for the dead baby, *"assuring them that ambivalence, overconcern and feelings of guilt or failure are quite normal"* (Cuisinier *et al.*, 1996, p. 343).
- **Encourage ritual.** Rituals can help families begin a healthy grief as well as celebrating the life, no matter how short it was. One of the first rituals that a pastoral care giver may be called upon to perform is a baptism or blessing of the dead baby. One pastoral care giver describes his experience of being called to the delivery room and asked to baptize a stillborn child:

  "The mother, father and I spoke softly, stood quietly and shared a moment of horror. I stroked her hair ... The parents would need to grieve the loss of their baby just like the death of any child. But before they could say good-bye, they had to have a way to say hello. Baptism is the moment in which the community of faith says 'Hello.' I began to understand more. One of the most important elements of the baptism is the naming. That name generates power that says 'this is a real person' ... With the full authority of my office, I told them that they must bury the baby and that we would have a graveside service. This baby would not disappear but have a proper place in history so that we could say 'Good-bye.'"
  Hanna Lothrop (1997, pp. 206–207)

- How meaningful such a ritual can be for grieving parents and family members! It is important to call the baby by name or say something like "your baby" if there is no name. Similarly, Eileen Connell encourages naming, as well as blessing and memorializing. Touch is also important. Sometimes family members of anyone who has died, not just a baby, are unsure if they should touch the corpse. As a pastoral care giver, you can model for them that it is okay to do so. Rituals do not have to be formal, such as a baptism or funeral; they can be very informal, such as touching and holding. There is nothing that should be considered frightening about a tiny baby. To deny a ritual for a grieving family can be a devastating blow, negating the loss. The following insight was experienced by Robert H. Loewy, a grieving father, and cited in Lothrop, 1997:

  "To deny ritual acknowledgment communicates the message that the family's loss is not at all significant, and that their baby was not a real person."
  Robert H. Loewy (cited in Lothrop, 1997, p. 208)

- It is especially important for faith communities to discover ways of honoring the life of a baby, even if he or she was born dead or miscarried. If no funeral was held, a memorial service could be held, even if years have elapsed. Another option might be acknowledging perinatal losses along with living babies at baby dedications on Mother's Day, for example. Presenting mothers with a rose in a worship service or a written announcement acknowledging the birth/death is another option. This would be done in a manner similar to announcing and recognizing the birth of a healthy baby.

- As stated at the outset, rituals for perinatal losses frequently occur in hospitals, but this was not always the case, as Diane Carroll relates:

  "A generation ago, hospitals whisked stillborns from their parents with a let's-forget-this-happened attitude. Now they encourage patients to spend time with their babies, creating the only face-to-face memories they will have."
  Diane Carroll (1996, p. 1)

- It is true that some parents or family, at least initially, will resist the opportunity of a face-to-face encounter with the dead baby. In fact, some family members may actively encourage the parents to resist, saying: "It will be much easier if you do not hold the baby." Such counsel is to be respected by the pastoral care giver. However, alternative options can also be offered. "I will be with you if you want to see the baby. I have seen her. She has a full head of hair. Would you like to see and hold her?" Even better, though, is to say, "My experience has shown that seeing, touching, holding, and naming your baby is very helpful."
- Additionally, some hospitals prepare packets of information for perinatal loss survivors. For example, pictures are taken; impressions of handprints or footprints may be taken; a lock of hair may be clipped. These can be important tangible reminders that the baby was real. Another consideration for remembering a ritual observance is to audio- or video-tape it. For grieving parents, almost everything surrounding the horrific experience of the loss is a blur, even the ritual. In cases of death, especially untimely deaths, the healthcare team and pastoral care givers have direct impact upon the family's emotional and spiritual well-being, an observation articulated by Brown and Sefansky:

  "Although little information is absorbed by parents at the time of a child's death, they remember the way they were treated by the healthcare team."
  Brown and Sefansky (1995, p. 59)

- Rituals at the funeral home can be helpful as well. The parents can be offered the opportunity to bathe, dress, and powder their baby. Photographs can be taken of the baby alone and as a member of the family—parents, siblings, grandparents. This final "little vehicle of parenting and being a family" can be valuable in the healing from the loss.
- Rituals (both formal and informal, in word and deed, performed by healthcare professionals or pastoral care givers, in the hospital or outside the hospital), are of utmost importance in facilitating healthy grief for parents who have experienced perinatal loss.
- **Administer grace.** An important role for pastoral care givers is to help the parents explore and sort through any feelings of guilt (Limbo *et al.*, 1986). People must talk about their guilt, or assumed guilt, to someone before they can find freedom in forgiveness: forgiveness of self. Give people permission to experience everything that is part of the grief journey, even a feeling of helplessness. It may be of tremendous help to them to accept such if the pastoral care giver is willing to admit his or her helplessness as well (Lothrop, 1997). One reason for helplessness is that the death of a child is absurd; children are not supposed to die (Miles, 1995). The administration of grace comes through nonjudgmental listening, providing caring instruction and sometimes confrontation, acknowledging the

baby's death, and affirming the right to grieve. Al Miles (1995) offers some advice for pastoral care givers as mediators of grace:

> *''Remember to reach out to the family instead of waiting for them to contact you ... We play a key role in supporting these families. Our compassionate, sensitive presence can help such families face the reality of death.''*
>
> *Al Miles (1995, pp. 39–40)*

- **Recommend a support group.** Even with the support of family, friends, a faith community and competent pastoral care providers, the bereaved parents may still struggle in comprehending the "what and the whys" of the experience. According to Lothrop (1997) no one understands bereaved parents like other bereaved parents. Those who are farther along in grief's journey can be helpful to those more recently bereaved. Therefore, one of the best things that a pastoral care giver can do is make a referral. However, the care giver should remain in the loop to offer any needed additional support.

So, what have we learned? Limbo *et al.* provide a succinct list of considerations for perinatal grievers, many of which were discussed in detail (1986, p. 140):

- seeing and holding the baby
- having private time
- making photographs
- receiving mementos
- discussing and planning funeral/memorial services
- having a baptism/blessing including the naming
- receiving information on the journey of grief.

Before concluding this, we want to say a word about another class of mothers—those who are unmarried. The grief they experience is no different and any less important than those of mothers with spouses. Their loss is just as real. They need support and validation for the experience of their losses. Pastoral care givers should not treat single mothers with any less dignity, respect, or compassion. The principles of care for those who grieve the loss of a baby can be applied to all without regard to any relationship affiliations or lack thereof.

One grieving mother eloquently and poignantly articulated the potency of perinatal loss:

> *''I doubt I will ever forget the babies I carried that were never born, and the power of that grief still catches me by surprise.''*
>
> *Citation in Bialosky and Schulman (1998, p. 79)*

5

When a Loved One Dies, Children Play and Cry

"Oh she is much too young to understand all of this." "Daddy's gone on a long trip." "Grandma went to sleep." Statements like these are commonly used by adults to explain to children the death of a family member or friend. Adults often want to shield children from death and grief. The prevalence of this is confirmed by Rosen's study of children and grief, with a special focus on sibling death (1984–85):

> *"The child is not given permission to remember the deceased or express feelings, but instead is encouraged to be strong and silent."*
>
> *Rosen (1984–85, p. 307)*

However, sooner or later, the shield is pulled away and children come face to face with death.

One thing is certain: children are not immune to death, particularly the deaths of close family members. One in twenty American children loses one or both parents to death—particularly in lower-income families; a higher percentage lose other relatives, neighbors, and friends (Parachin, 2006, p. 60). Dr. Sherwin B. Nuland's childhood encounter with death convinced him that loss is life shaping and a determinant of how he or she (and the adult he or she becomes) deals with death:

> *"My mother died of colon cancer one week after my eleventh birthday, and that fact has shaped my life. All that I have become and much that I have not become, I trace directly or indirectly to her death."*
>
> *Dr. Sherwin B. Nuland (2003, p. xviii)*

Nuland became a prominent surgeon at Yale Medical School and a prize-winning author for the book *How We Die*. Had his mother not died when she did, would that have changed the course of his life?

This chapter addresses issues of children grieving the loss of a loved one or friends through death. Speece and Brent (1996) have identified death-related concepts, which, when understood, can better enable a person's adjustment to the permanent absence of a loved one (*see* Box 5.1).

Box 5.1	
Universality:	All living things die.
Inevitability:	Everyone, including you, will die.
Irreversibility:	This is a difficult concept for children to understand since they see people die on television, who reappear elsewhere alive.
Unpredictability:	Anyone can die at any time.

Nonfunctionality:	This is also difficult for children to understand, that nothing about the body "works" anymore.
Causality:	The medical explanation for death may not translate into a child's experience. Rather, children themselves may assume responsibility. "Because I was bad ..." or "Because I didn't obey, mommy died." "It was my fault."
Noncorporeality:	"Where is Daddy now?"

As important as these concepts are to comprehend intellectually, it is far more important that they be understood experientially. Therefore, key components in the shaping of children's initial experience with death are the circumstances of the death, the resulting changes in the child's living environment, and the adult responses around them. Corr (in Corr *et al.*, 1997) identifies three additional factors which significantly impact children's grief experiences:

1. personality of the child
2. child's ability/inability to communicate what is being experienced
3. things which the situational environment (circumstances, familial/cultural traditions, etc.) does or does not permit.

More recently, Corr (2000) builds upon his previous work of fleshing out the realities which mold a child's encounter with death:

- Children often lack prior experience with such strong and hard-to-understand reactions from adults.
- Children often lack the conceptual ability to label and understand what they are experiencing.
- Children often lack the communicative skills with which to articulate their grief reactions.

Because of the existence of these realities with respect to children and grief, Krietemeyer and Heirey (1992) suggest a three-fold purpose for response to grieving children:

1. Help the child to put the event into perspective.
2. Help the child make sense of the confusion—both the death and the confusion of adults with the death.
3. Help the child begin to develop an understanding of this death and death in general.

The method they use and endorse is storytelling. On the other hand, Nancy Webb (2000) uses play therapy as a vehicle to help the child process what is happening in a safe manner.

> *"Children in play use dolls, drawings, games, and other toys as shields that protect them from admitting that frightening things have happened to them and may still be happening to them."*
>
> *Nancy Webb (2000, p. 141)*

Play therapy gives a grieving child two things (Webb, 2000, p. 141):

1. a place to maintain a comfort zone of distance between the content of the play and his or her own situation
2. a safe disguise which permits the child to express anger, jealousy, and fear through the mouths of puppets or dolls.

In addition Mufson *et al.* suggest that four frameworks of reference should be assessed in order to more accurately determine death's impact on children: both present and future (1993, pp. 90–91):

1. child's role in the family system or peer group before and after the death
2. child's psychological maturity and coping skills at the time of the crisis
3. child's remaining social and familial support network
4. nature of the relationship ended by death.

Death impacts children. The degree to which it has negative lingering effects falls squarely upon the shoulders of the adults in the sphere of influence. Noted grief scholar Robert Kastenbaum (2000) contends:

> *"We can be more useful to children ... if we can share with them realities as well as fantasies about death. This means some uncomfortable moments. Part of each child's adventure into life is the discovery of loss, separation, nonbeing, and death. No one else can have this experience for the child, nor can death be locked into another room until a child comes of age."*
>
> Robert Kastenbaum (2000, pp. 19–20)

Attempting to soften the impact of death upon children and continually shield them from its reality through fantasy and storybook tales is much easier for adults or older siblings. In fact, it is only natural to protect the very young from horrific events. However, to do so repeatedly without introducing serious realities can impair healthy grief.

Therefore, since it is a given that children, even the youngest who may not fully comprehend what has happened, grieve, what are the tasks associated with that process? Baker, Sedney, and Gross (1992) identify six:

1. **Understanding that someone has died**: The word "died," although brutal in a certain sense, is an essential component of communication if the child is to understand that the deceased is not simply asleep. This concept can be confusing for children who did not have daily or regular contact with the deceased. The child may think (or pretend) he or she is away on a trip.
2. **Protecting self and significant others**: *"A very bad man kilt him!"* was one child's explanation of a kidnapped peer's death. The child then asked, *"Will that bad man get me or my brother?"* Children need to understand that, in the vast majority of cases, one event which causes them pain is not a concern for fear that the same thing will happen to them. They need constant reassurance of that fact.
3. **Accepting and emotionally acknowledging the loss**: Unfortunately, many adults expect children to grieve like little adults. However, in reality, children grieve quite differently. On the one hand, children may exhibit "expected" grief symptoms. On the other, they may play by themselves or with friends, seemingly oblivious to the fact that "death" has occurred. Adults must understand this and allow children to accept the loss in their own ways.

4. **Facing and bearing the pain**: Many individuals desire to limit a child's exposure to painful experiences resulting from a death. For example, people may not allow children to view the deceased's body, go to the funeral or attend any burial or scattering ceremony. In a good many cases, these attempts to protect children from facing the reality of what happened can prolong or delay grief. Even young children who do not understand any of the rituals can be told about them later as a way of helping them to understand more fully what happened.

5. **Exploring and re-evaluating the relationship to the deceased**: How does a child understand the ramifications of a dead father, mother (or both), sibling, or close friend? What was the quality of the relationship? How will the absence of that person in a child's life affect the child, immediately and long-term? These, among others, are questions for reflection in evaluating a child's well-being following the death of a parent, care-giving close relative, or friend.

6. **Coping with the future**: Death changes the environment in one's home. This is especially true for children who are dependent in some ways upon the deceased. For children, the death of a parent, a sibling, a friend, or a beloved grandparent presents the strong possibility of a physical, emotional, or spiritual crisis. The physical crisis could be refusing to eat, potentially harmful behavior, etc. The emotional crisis could be mood swings or serious depression. The spiritual crisis could result in resentment against God, which could continue into adulthood. Some well-meaning person told one little girl, "God wanted her little sister because she was so good." She responded: "Then I am going to be bad so he won't take me, too." All adults must be careful what they say. Now, any of these three crises may happen with children, and some may go unnoticed because a physically present but emotionally absent grieving parent may be so deep in his or her own grief. Therefore, other adults and older siblings need to be aware that these potential crises exist and, thus, be watchful. In so doing and intervening if any of them arises, a child's ability to cope in the present and future is greatly enhanced.

Should children be included in the rituals surrounding death? Funeral director Eric Voide says, yes. In the article "Children Should Be Seen and Heard," he states that the "inclusion of a child will serve to demystify the process and aid in future dealings with death" (1998, p. 28). Voide concedes, though, that children's attendance at funerals or memorial services should never be forced. Certainly, children have a natural curiosity about death. They play doctor, nurse, patient. They play games: "Bang you're dead." Joy Johnson states that, prior to the funeral ritual, children can be included. For example, children can place a stuffed animal or toy in the casket, help decide what clothes to choose for the deceased, bring a favorite object belonging to the deceased to hold during the service. They could also do a drawing or make a card which could be placed in the casket or given to another griever.

If death cannot be hidden from children, why should rituals be hidden? Before making the decisions not to involve children in death rituals, Kenneth Doka offers practical suggestions for preparing a child for participation (2000, pp. 155–156):

- Explain to children what a visitation, funeral, and committal are and what is likely to happen during those rituals.
- Describe the purpose of the rituals.
- Describe the physical settings where the rituals will occur.

- Describe the various ways in which people may behave (e.g. faint abruptly and loudly leave).
- Explain that some individuals may cry.
- Explain that some people may laugh.
- Give children time to talk and think about the decision to participate.
- Give children the option not to attend or leave once they are there.
- Give the child something to do in the ritual.

Doka also suggests that someone should be designated as a support person for children at the death rituals because the parent(s) may be so overcome with grief that they may be unable to be attentive to the children. A child can get emotionally and physically lost at a ritual. Johnson suggests that children can have their own viewing of the deceased, along with time for questions.

With respect to funeral planning, a Kansas City, Missouri faith congregation includes some information regarding children in *A Guide to Funeral Planning at Saint Francis Xavier*:

> *"Parents need to prepare the child for the service by explaining what will happen and why."*
>
> Saint Francis Xavier Church (1996, p. 4)

That is good advice. Another consideration is to introduce children to rituals when a pet dies. To make good decisions when death comes in a child's life and decisions about rituals, children need the following:

- information
- options
- support.

Doka concurs with this counsel:

> *"Since funerals are so critical, once children are developmentally able to understand a funeral and sit through a ceremony, they ought to have a choice about the ways in which they wish to participate in a funeral."*
>
> Kenneth Doka (2000, p. 155)

Beyond those initial concerns concerning rituals, what are the bereavement needs of children? William Worden has identified a number of factors to consider (1996, pp. 140–146):

- age-appropriate information about the death
- fears and anxieties addressed
- reassurance that they are not to blame for the death—"I was bad, so Mommy died."
- careful listening by others to what is and is not said
- validation of feelings—to be sad, confused, indifferent, etc.
- help processing and dealing with feelings that overwhelm
- involvement and inclusion
- continuation of routine activities
- modeled grief behaviors— "How should I act?"
- permission and opportunities to remember, especially critical if a child concludes that remembering makes another family member sad.

"Loss hurts, and we cannot find the words to soothe that hurt—there aren't any. We cannot shield our children from the twists and turns of living. We cannot protect them from experiencing life (and death). We can, however, build supports and safety nets, not only for our children, but for ourselves as well.

"Hurt and pain have their lessons, and we cannot rob our children of the richness of the tapestry that hurt and love weave together."

Darcie Sims (1991, p. 189)

How profound are those words! *"... we cannot rob our children of the richness ..."* How can people help children experience the richness of what is otherwise a time of sorrow? The following is a list of things that individuals can do to help children grieve in a healthy manner:

- Avoid euphemisms (e.g. "Your daddy or (name of person) went to sleep").
- Listen all of the way to the end of their sentences, even those which ramble.
- Listen with your ears and your eyes.
- Bend or kneel down or pick up the child in order to facilitate dialogue.
- Let a child's natural curiosity create discussions. "We'll talk about that later" may send a message that such a subject is taboo.
- Be open to and value a child's wonderings: "Will he still go fishing?"
- Do not take over or stifle a child's expressions of feelings: "Stop crying!" Or "Big girls don't cry."
- Reassure the child of your active presence in his or her life: "I am here for you."
- Allow "time outs" for playing.
- Actively include the child in rituals.
- Encourage familiar routines: regular mealtimes, bed at the appropriate time, etc. (i.e. as much as possible in what is an otherwise chaotic time).
- Ask the child to describe favorite memories. Prompt responses by, for example, "Do you remember the time we went to Disney World and ...?"
- Help the child create a memory that can be cherished. For some children, given an abusive relationship with the deceased, this may be difficult.
- Be conscious of the child's eating habits. Limit junk food. Plan well-balanced meals.
- Be aware that going back to school may be healthy as a safe place to grieve and receive nurture. Make sure that teacher(s) know of the death.
- Give boys permission to grieve; some boys express their grief better if you sit beside instead of facing them.
- Look for "discounted" grievers. Some parents may think the child is too young to really know what is going on and say, "Oh, he will be fine."
- Find ways to help the child remember holidays and other special days, especially birthdays.
- Remember that you do not need to protect or defend God from a child's anger.
- Grant children the freedom to cry. Hold them tightly, but touch appropriately.
- Pray for and with the child. Listen to the child's prayer.
- Attend rituals as a support person for the child. Seeing a familiar face can be enormously helpful.
- Offer to accompany a child to the cemetery or scattering area after the rituals.
- Do not be too quick to offer easy answers.

- Do not attempt to distract the child from grief work through activities and busy-ness.
- Do not encourage the child to ''get over'' the loss.
- Take any suicide threat seriously. Children can complete suicide.
- Know competent resources for referral.
- Be alert to warning signals of distress.
- Learn locations of centers for grieving children.
- Learn how to explain disposition of the body (i.e. burial, cremation, etc.)
- Contact The Centering Corporation, the largest distributors of resources for grieving children (resources both in English and Spanish). www.centering.org

What are some warning signals of which to be conscious that might indicate the need for professional help? Worden offers ten for consideration (1996, pp. 147–149):

1. persistent difficulty talking about the deceased
2. aggressive behavior (kicking, biting, hitting)
3. persistent anxiety
4. persistent somatic (i.e. bodily) complaints
5. persistent sleeping difficulties
6. persistent self-blame or guilt
7. eating disturbances
8. marked social withdrawal
9. serious academic reversal
10. self-destructive behavior.

Any statement such as ''I wish I could die and go be with [name of person]'' should be taken seriously.

Why do children need support of others and possibly even professional help after the death of a significant loved one? Kooten and Flowers answer:

> *''These younger persons are being forced to deal with a major life issue long before they are emotionally and experientially ready for it, and the level of terror and anxiety they feel can seem out of proportion to the threat.''*
>
> *Kooten and Flowers (2000, p. 301)*

Joy Johnson (2006) believes that children can deal with grief as well as, and sometimes better than, adults when they are given love and support. She goes on to say that ''we've learned that children will hold onto their grief until they see adults around them grieving in a healthy way and know they are safe to grieve too.''

Throughout this chapter, we have discussed grief related to the physical death of a loved one. Mahan (1999) calls attention to the fact that a death may precipitate other losses. For example, if the death(s) cause a child to become an orphan, the child not only loses his parents (or whomever he or she lives with) but perhaps a home, a school, friends, playgrounds, and familiar routines. Sometimes, children from the same family are split up. Hence, not only did a child lose parents or guardians, but siblings as well. Moreover, the parent may be so incapacitated by grief that they are unavailable to their children; in some cases, the child has become the parent. Famed tennis great, Arthur Ashe, then age six, told his father after his mother's death, ''Don't cry Daddy. As long as we have each other, we'll be all right'' (Ashe and McCabe, 1995, p. 50).

"Death is never easy. This is especially true for children whose world can be turned upside down."

SLJ

Sooner or later, children will encounter life's great lessons on death. Nancy Crump suggests this about children and grief:

"A significant element in children grieving in a healthy manner is how well the adults in their lives are grieving."

Nancy Crump

Finally, the ultimate goal of care givers for children who have lost a loved one through death (or some other type of physical separation) is to provide a safe, caring, comfortable atmosphere in which they can grapple with and express their feelings about the loss and learn about the journey of grief. Put these words of Baker, Sedney, and Gross into your memory bank:

"Even in the best circumstances, the grief process in children will extend for many years after the time of death."

Baker, Sedney, and Gross (1992, p. 114)

6

Adolescents: Grief's In-Between Generation

The stage of adolescence itself can be quite a challenge for all who pass through it. Part of this challenge involves repeated attempts at answering two questions:

1. Who am I?
2. What am I?

Adolescence is a time of ambivalence, not only for teens, but also for their parents and other adults with whom they interact. Therese Rando has some salient words to say, especially to adults, concerning this confusing period of time in a person's life:

> *"Recognize that the adolescent is half child and half adult. Do not treat her (or him) as too much of either one or the other."*
>
> *Therese Rando (1984, p. 413)*

At this stage in their lives, which we might describe as the "land in-between," adolescents are searching for meaning, identity, relationships. If a death of a family member, friend or schoolmate is added to the mix of an already complicated life, a teen's ability to cope can be seriously impaired. One thing is certain, teens, like everyone else, are not immune to the reality of death.

One study of 1,000 high school juniors and seniors revealed that 90% of those surveyed had experienced the death of someone they loved and 40% had lost a friend or peer whose age was in close proximity to their own (Ewalt and Perkins, 1979). Readers will find this latter statistic alarming: 40% had experienced the loss of a peer through death. Even though this study is somewhat dated, more recent studies confirm that this trend is continuing at an increasing rate. Note carefully the number of adolescent deaths in 1996 reflected in Tables 6.1 and 6.2 (U.S. Census Bureau, 1999, p. 101).

Table 6.1   Death of Adolescents 10–19 Years of Age (Total 19,300)

Accidents/adverse effects	8,600
Homicide/legal intervention	3,100
Suicide	2,100

The statistics become more shocking when we look at a different age range, one more often used by "suicidologists" and researchers (*see* Table 6.2).

Table 6.2   Death of Adolescents 15–24 Years of Age (Total 32,500)

Accidents/adverse effects	13,900
Homicide/legal intervention	4,300
Suicide	6,500

The percentage of deaths from unnatural causes in Table 6.1 is 70%; the percentage of deaths from unnatural causes in Table 6.2 is 76%. Some might question the inclusion of people in their twenties in the second grid. Arguably for many, the early twenties is an extension of adolescence because significant numbers of teens know and associate with people in that age bracket. That is most likely the major reason researchers typically group death statistics according to this framework. It is also quite possible that the awareness of these startling numbers is the precipitating factor for the outcry of Etienne Krug (in Center for Disease Control, 1998):

> *''Our children are getting killed or killing themselves at higher rates than any other country. No child should die a violent death in the most industrialized country in the world.''*
> *Etienne Krug (in Murder, Suicide Taking More of U.S. Youths, p. A.9)*

Unfortunately, adolescents' grief is often discounted to the degree that Balk (1991) calls them the ''forgotten'' grievers. Nancy Crump broadens Balk's assessment to include all children as forgotten grievers. Cook and Oltjenbruns (1998) suggest that this is particularly the case when a boyfriend/girlfriend or an ''ex'' dies, especially if others did not sanction the relationship. Furthermore, in cases of violent (intentional or accidental) deaths, teenagers may experience survivor guilt asking questions like the following:

- ''Why wasn't I with them the night of the accident?''
- ''Why was I spared?''
- ''Why did I live?''

As a result of wrestling with these unanswerable questions along with the perception that their grief does not count, Rando states that adolescents may act out in ''care-eliciting'' behaviors.

Concerning the nature of adolescence and grief, Raphael (1983) has identified feelings they commonly experience:

- sadness about having to cope with the loss of the relationship
- excessive guilt regarding activities they wish they had or had not done with the deceased
- anger at being left behind
- remorse over not having had the chance to say good-bye
- responsibility, that perhaps if they had done something different, the deceased would still be with them
- concern that the same thing may happen again to someone else or to them
- over-identification with the deceased in order to maintain continuity of presence.

Crump enumerates other concerns that children have:

- ''Who will take me to ball practice?''
- ''Who will take me to dance lessons?''
- ''What will happen to me now?''

Similarly, Carole Staudacher highlights several, what she calls, ''stereotypical'' male adolescent grief responses (1991):

- withdrawal and stifling emotions
- substituting anger and aggression for other feelings

- maintaining silence (or minimal responses to questions)
- repressing feelings of guilt
- experiencing confusion.

Related to these are what Worden (1996) cites as core issues which adolescents whose lives are impacted by death typically face:

- predictability of events
- development of self-image
- sense of fairness and justice
- mastery and control.

In order to assess more appropriately the feelings (Raphael), the response (Staudacher), and the core issues (Worden), all of which determine the impact of a death on an adolescent, Mufson *et al.* state that four frameworks of concern be considered: these were the same four as mentioned previously in the discussion of grieving children (1993, pp. 90–91):

1. Teen's role and place in the family system or peer group before and after the death. (When a sibling dies, the order changes. In one day, Ben became the oldest brother when his older brother was murdered.)
2. Nature of the relationship lost.
3. Remaining social and familial support network.
4. Teen's psychological maturity and coping skills at the time of the death.

Furthermore, it is also important in assessing the impact of a death on adolescents to be aware of certain assumptions regarding teens and loss through death. Neimeyer has suggested the following (1998, p. 109):

- Loss as an event can validate or invalidate the assumptions and values by which a teen lives.
- For example, adolescents often feel invincible: "Things happen, but not to me." "I can drink and drive and not die." "I can do drugs and not overdose." A death of a close peer who died as a result of an alcohol- or other drug-related incident can provide a significant "wake-up call" because a life assumption has now been proven invalid.
- Grieving is the act of affirming or reconstructing a personal world of meaning that has been challenged by loss.
- Grieving teens adapt to loss by restoring coherence to the narratives of their lives.
- Teens do not ever get over a peer's death or the death of a parent or sibling, but they can come to some sense of peace with the loss.
- Grieving teens construct and reconstruct their identities as survivors in negotiation with others.
- Teens will ask questions like these: "Why?" "Why her?" "Why not me?" "Why now?" The key question is to whom will they ask those questions? That person may be a parent, other adult, or peer. Over time, the individuals to whom questions are addressed may change for any number of reasons. The teen may marry and the safe person to ask questions of is now the spouse.
- Grieving is something that adolescents do, not something that is done for them.
- There is a temptation to want to rescue a young teen from his or her encounter with grief or attempt to somehow make it up to the teen for what has been experienced.
- Grief is a personal process: individual, intimate and inescapable.

After becoming aware of the items addressed by Raphael, Worden, and Neimeyer in the preceding pages, what are some things that an individual can do to help adolescents grieve in a healthy manner? The following list of practical suggestions can be effectively used to accomplish that purpose.

- Avoid clichés.
- Listen all of the way to the end of their sentences, even those which ramble.
- Give the teen permission to say the deceased's name aloud and to tell stories about the individual or their relationship.
- Keep confidences.
- Look for discounted grievers; remember, adolescents are what Balk calls the "forgotten" grievers.
- Let teens cry.
- Give males permission to grieve. Sit beside them to talk or do "car therapy." Take a ride.
- Ask who is giving them advice.
- Pray for and with the grieving teen.
- Discourage hasty decisions.
- Be conscious of their eating habits and encourage healthy eating.
- Remember that you do not need to protect or defend God from an adolescent's anger.
- Applaud "baby steps" in reconciling with the loss.
- Help an adolescent acknowledge the good and the bad in the deceased.
- Find a way to help the grieving adolescent remember and "make special."
- Attend rituals as a support person for the grieving adolescent.
- Consider doing a good deed in the name of the deceased, particularly something that the deceased would have done.
- Be alert to the grief "numb-ers:" alcohol, drugs, risky behaviors, etc.
- Encourage the adolescent to do the "hard time" with grief.
- Remember that the death of a peer the adolescent does not know is still a significant blow (e.g. a fellow student killed in an auto accident affects an entire school).
- Do not be too quick with easy answers; listen carefully to the asked and unasked questions.
- Do not encourage the adolescent to get over the loss.
- Do not attempt to distract the teen from grief work through activities.
- Take any suicide threat seriously.
- Know good sources for referral.
- Be alert to warning signals of distress.

However, even if thorough assessment has taken place, problem areas are identified and appropriate support made available, some grieving adolescents may still be having difficulty and need extra help. Wolfelt has identified warning signals of grieving adolescents who need that extra help. Parachin (1998b, May, 16) has identified warning signals of grieving adolescents who need that extra help:

- Appetite changes resulting in dramatic weight gain or loss.
- Altered sleep patterns—either unable to rest or sleeping excessively.
- Prolonged withdrawal from others.
- Deterioration of relationships with family and friends.

- Risk-taking behaviors such as drug and alcohol abuse or
- sexual experimentation.
- Inability to experience pleasure.
- Feeling overly guilty, hostile or resentful.
- Demonstrating helplessness and hopelessness.

Finally, the goal of pastoral care with adolescents is to assure them that their grief counts; they are not forgotten in the circle of those grieving the loss. Additionally, they, like all other grievers, need a safe place to express their feelings, share their concerns and to learn about the grief journey. Above all else, when providing pastoral care to a grieving adolescent, remember these words of Neimeyer:

> *"One's world is forever transformed by loss."*
>
> *Neimeyer (1998, p. 86)*

7

Men and Women: Do They Grieve the Same?

No two people grieve the same; a person's grief print and thumbprint are both unique. Interestingly, though, women are often regarded as the gender-specific group who grieve "correctly" or who have societal permission to grieve more emotionally. Therefore, the issue of male grievers of all ages has been a topic of great concern among pastoral care givers and grief specialists, particularly Terry Martin and Kenneth Doka. Contemplate their words reflecting the perceived differences between men and women as grievers:

> *"In grief, we treat males the way we treat females in many other contexts—we judge them according to what is normal for the other sex. In truth, the mosaic of behaviors deemed 'normal grief' is primarily based on samples of women. When men are evaluated against these norms, they are judged as grieving not as 'well' or as 'completely.'"*
>
> Martin and Doka (1996, pp. 161–162)

In 1997, Eugene McDowell and a group of colleagues reported the results of their study of certified grief counselors' and grief therapists' perspectives on gender differences in grief ("Women's Issues in Grief." Paper presented at the annual meeting of the Association for Death Education and Counseling, Washington, DC, 1997). The researchers found that the participants in their sample believed that women and men express grief differently. Men were perceived as less likely to express strong emotions and more likely to use diversions such as work, play, sex, or alcohol. Therapists reported that men were more likely to respond cognitively and to use anger as a primary mode of emotional expression. Women were seen as more likely to express grief affectively (emotionally) and to seek support.

The perspective of these therapists, explicitly or implicitly, is grounded in much of the research that does show a difference in the ways men and women grieve. In summarizing this research in 1999, Terry Martin and Kenneth J. Doka (1996) noted:

1. Research has shown that widows and widowers face different problems in grief. For example, many widows reported financial distress and noted the emotional support that had been provided by their spouse. Widowers were more likely to report disruptions of their familial and social networks. Widows were more likely to seek emotional support, whereas widowers found solace in exercise, work, religion, creative expression, or more destructively in alcohol.
2. Many of these same results are evident following the death of a child. Mothers reported more emotional distress than fathers. Strategies in dealing with the loss differed by gender. Women tended to use more support-seeking and emotion-

focused strategies, whereas men were more likely to intellectualize their grief and use more problem-focused strategies to adapt to the loss.

3. Studies of the loss of a parent also showed that middle-aged sons were less likely than daughters to experience intense grief, had fewer physical manifestations of grief, and were more likely to use cognitive and active approaches in adapting to loss.

4. Differences between genders seem less apparent in older age groups. This may reflect the idea that individuals become more androgynous as they age.

5. Differences in gender are also affected by other variables such as social class, generational differences, and cultural differences.

6. The research on differences in outcome is quite mixed. Some studies have shown men to have better outcomes, others show women to do better, and still other studies show no significant difference or mixed results in outcome (i.e. men do better on some measures, women on other measures).

While it is important for both sexes to grieve healthily, there is the pervasive myth that men grieve in a manner far less healthy than women. Martin's and Doka's 2000 work *Men Don't Cry, Women Do: Transcending Gender Stereotypes on Grief* challenges this popular notion that men are "poor grievers" when compared against women. Or the notion: "Women grieve/men replace." They suggest pastoral care givers look beyond gender to understand different patterns or styles of grief and propose that these patterns are related to gender but not determined by it. They further suggested that gender, culture, and initial temperament all interact to produce a dominant pattern of grief. They viewed these patterns of grief as a continuum. They also acknowledged that patterns are likely to change throughout an individual's development, often moving more toward the center of the continuum as an individual moves to late adulthood. Based upon the underlying concept of emotion regulation, Martin and Doka proposed three basic patterns of grief: intuitive, instrumental, and dissonant.

- *Intuitive pattern.* Intuitive grievers experience, express, and adapt to grief on a very affective level. Intuitive grievers are likely to report the experience of grief as waves of affect, or feeling. They are likely to strongly express these emotions as they grieve—shouting, crying, or displaying emotion in other ways. Intuitive grievers are also likely to be helped in ways that allow them to ventilate their emotions. Self-help and support groups, counseling, and other expressive opportunities that allow these grievers to ventilate feelings are likely to be helpful.

- *Instrumental pattern.* Instrumental grievers are more likely to experience, express, and adapt to grief in more active and cognitive ways. Instrumental grievers will tend to experience grief as thoughts, such as a flooding of memories, or in physical or behavioral manifestations. They are likely to express grief in similar ways—doing something related to the loss, exercising, or talking about the loss. For example, in one case, a man whose daughter died in a car crash found great solace in repairing the fence his daughter had wrecked. "It was," he shared later, "the only part of the accident I could fix" (Martin and Doka, 2000). Instrumental grievers are helped by strategies such as the use of self-help literature and other interventions that make use of cognitive and active approaches.

- *Dissonant pattern.* Dissonant grievers are those who experience grief in one pattern but who are inhibited from ways to express or adapt to grief that are compatible with their experience. For example, a man might experience grief intuitively but feel constrained from expressing or adapting to grief in that way because he perceives it as inimical to his male role. Similarly, a woman might also experience grief in a more intuitive way but believe she has to repress that feeling in order to protect her family. Counseling with dissonant grievers involves helping to identify their inherent pattern, recognizing the barriers to effective expression and adaptation, and developing suitable intervention techniques.

Some of the material related in the preceding paragraphs about "styles of grief" was extracted from a paper by Ken Doka entitled "Gender" (www.deathreference.com/Gi-Ho/Grief.html). Doka also related to me (SLJ) in a personal memorandum: "These styles simply represent differences in the way people grieve and not deficiencies. Persons (men and women) of different styles experience, express and adapt to loss in distinct ways."

Where are men and women found on this continuum? Martin and Doka suggested that many men, at least in Western culture, are likely to be found on the instrumental end of this continuum whereas women are more likely to be found on the intuitive end. The researchers stressed, however, that while gender does influence the pattern of grief, that pattern is not determined by gender. Martin and Doka also noted that many individuals in the center of the continuum may show more blended patterns, using a range of emotional, behavioral, and cognitive strategies to adapt to loss. Moreover, they might respond to a particular death in one manner, and in another manner to another death.

Other grief specialists contend that grief patterns are more gender related or gender determined. Their views should not be summarily dismissed. This chapter will introduce material from the differing viewpoints. The authors will argue, though, that what is perceived by some as male-specific grief expressions can also be (and often is) characteristic of grieving women and vice versa, reflecting the notion of the influence of styles rather simply gender.

What, then, are some general assumptions about grieving men when compared with grieving women? Martin and Doka have identified seven (1996, pp. 167–168):

1. Feelings are controlled.
2. Thinking precedes and often dominates feelings.
3. Focus may be on problem-solving rather than expression of feelings.
4. Outward expression of feelings often involves anger and/or guilt. (The latter is often true with women.)
5. Internal adjustments to the loss usually are expressed through activity.
6. Intense grief usually is expressed immediately after the loss, often during post-death rituals. (This is equally true for women.)
7. Intense feelings are experienced privately.

In *Men and Grief: A Guide for Men Surviving the Death of a Loved One* (1991), Carol Staudacher discusses several things related to male grief, which are somewhat different from female grief. The reality is, though, that a number of the items listed address grief issues of both sexes.

How a male will grieve a particular loss is, according to Staudacher, influenced by several factors (1991, p. 69):

- number of losses sustained up to the point of the present loss
- how the person has dealt (or is dealing) with grief from earlier losses
- amount and type of support available to the person.

All of these indicators are key components in determining how men and women grieve a particular loss. Concerning the last one, support may be difficult for many men to receive. Even when support is readily available, convincing many males to admit "needing" support may be a difficult task.

Additionally, Staudacher identifies several feelings men commonly experience in bereavement (1991, p. 84):

- feeling abandoned
- feeling closer to death themselves
- feeling frustrated
- feeling relieved and released
- feeling vulnerable.

Once again, both men and women experience all of these feelings to some degree. In fact, women may experience feeling financially vulnerable to a greater level of intensity, especially if the man was the primary "bread winner" in the home. Similarly, Staudacher suggests that a male griever may experience certain fears (1991, p. 148):

- fear of being vulnerable
- fear of being misunderstood
- fear of hurting other survivors
- fear of losing control
- fear of losing the respect or admiration of others.

And the male may fear being identified as "weak." Of these fears and the previously listed feelings, there are none that could or should be designated as exclusive to male grievers. While men and women may experience and express the same feelings (abandoned, frustrated, etc.) and fears (vulnerability, losing control, etc.) differently, nevertheless they are living with the same feelings and fears. However, the fear of losing the respect or admiration of others is, most assuredly, far more dominant in men. Why is this? The answer is related to instructions given to males:

- "Don't cry!"
- "Be strong!"
- "Get hold of yourself!"
- "Take it like a man!"
- "Big boys don't cry!"

Men have heard statements like these throughout their lives but particularly in childhood. Consequently, not crying, being strong, getting hold of yourself, "taking it like a man" proves that you are in control. Thus, you have, or gain, the respect of others for "taking it so well."

How inhibiting that mindset from cultural perception truly is.

- Real men do cry.
- Real men do not have to be strong.

Tim Madigan writes about his friendship with television personality [Mr.] Fred Rogers, particularly enhanced during the illness and death of Tim's brother, Steve. At the point he realized that Rogers' death was imminent he spent "the next four hours driving alone in the rural hills of North Texas, with sad music playing in my car, nearly blinded by the tears." Then Madigan, a Fort Worth newspaper reporter, wrote about his grief in a column in the *Star*. "Now Fred is gone and my heart is broken." He was inundated with telephone calls and emails from readers who wanted to share their stories and validate his public grieving for a friend (Madigan, 2006, pp. 186–187).

Staudacher confirms honest exploration and expression of grief:

> *"One of the most valuable sources of support a man can have following his loved one's death is the genuine friendship and companionship of another man or other men. A survivor may have the support and comfort of women, but within that nurturing friendship, regardless of how generous and intense it is, one special and important component is missing: the acceptance of the male survivor's grief-related behavior by another man."*
>
> Carol Staudacher (1991, p. 201)

Another area in which men are inhibited in grief is when they assume the role of grief manager. Some men, particularly fathers, initially respond to grief from a task-oriented perspective: What needs to be done? What has to be done? Martin and Doka quote one father whose 17-year-old son died: *"I couldn't allow myself to miss him, until I figured out what I needed to do to help our family deal with (his) death"* (1996, p. 163). These words are a reflection of the man's role as provider. A father also views himself in the role of protector, at least in the physical sense. Thus, if a child is killed, a typical fatherly response would be: "I shouldn't have let him go out that night." The father blames himself.

Similarly, women frequently assume the role of grief manager. When there are children in the close circle of grievers, mothers take charge orchestrating details and making arrangements in the attempt to provide some sense of normalcy for the family in the midst of a chaotic time. They become the protector of the family's emotions. In many circumstances, women also view themselves as provider. This is especially the case in single-parent homes. Therefore, it would not be uncommon to hear a mother say similar words to those cited by Martin and Doka in the previous paragraph.

Since men and women function as grief managers, the following statement of Staudacher applies equally to both:

> *"You not only manage your own grief, you may also try to manage others' grief as well. If so, your rationale may be that if you or others do or don't do certain things, the grief of your loved ones will be made easier or shorter."*
>
> Carol Staudacher (1991, p. 124)

There are situations in which the stress of grief may be overwhelming: for example, when someone is believed to be "at fault" or responsible for the death. In cases like these, both men and women must consider decisions seriously and cautiously because choices always have consequences: good and bad. The following is a list of some choices grieving adults may have to make in the aftermath of tragic, violent deaths.

- **Remain silent; be vocal.** "Anything you say or do can be used against you."
- **Defer to your spouse.** "Whatever you say" or "Whatever you think is best."
- **Engage in solitary mourning or secret grief.** In attempts to be strong (or to appear that way), men and/or women may discourage grief by other family members.

- **Take physical action.** "I'll get him for this!" is more of a typical male response than that of a female.
- **Investigate and take legal action.** In a litigious society, many adults immediately turn to the police and/or attorneys for prosecution of or to sue the "responsible" person.
- **Become immersed in activity.** "Stay busy" is one of the most common maxims in this society. Many grievers immediately get to work on details of settling an estate or cleaning out closets, possessions, etc.
- **Seek solace elsewhere.** If intimacy is not part of a couple's shared grief experience, one or both may look elsewhere for comfort from someone of the opposite sex.
- **Numb the pain.** Ironically, many can only express grief emotions when drinking or using some drug other than alcohol. For some "who have been sober," grief can be a significant challenge to that sobriety. Other "numb-ers" can be gambling, overeating, working long hours, etc.
- **Get over the loss rather than reconcile with it.** Typically, this is more of a male mentality.

We think it is obvious to most people that to say "yes" to the majority of the things presented would be to exhibit poor judgment. In some of the other cases (e.g. defer to the spouse, take physical action) thoughtful contemplation needs to precede any action taken. Consider the pros and cons for whatever action is being considered.

Not only is grief difficult when parents are left behind to grieve the loss of a child, whether through natural death or through unnatural death as discussed above, but also when a spouse who is also a best friend dies. This is a dual crisis, especially when there are no children or when children are grown and do not live at home.

- "We did everything together."
- "He/she is my life."
- "What will I do without him/her?"

These are not uncommon statements to hear from widows and widowers or unmarried partners. The death of a spouse is often a devastating blow to the surviving husband or wife, as described by Raphael:

> *"When the relationship with a partner is such that their lives are closely interwoven, the loss of one partner may cut across the very meaning of the other's existence."*
>
> Raphael (1983, p. 177)

These words of Corr, Nabe, and Corr complement Raphael's thinking:

> *"It appears that those who have experienced the death of a spouse or life partner are at a higher risk during the following year for increased morbidity and mortality."*
>
> Corr et al. (1997, p. 423)

Adult grief is especially hard. Victor M. Parachin offers wise advice for men in an article entitled, "The Mourning After: Ten Healing Steps for Grieving Men" (1998c, pp. 20, 22, 24). However, we believe his ten "gifts" of healing words apply to both men **and** women.

1. Expect and accept emotional turmoil.
2. Become informed about grief.

3. Commit to adapting and adjusting.
4. Adopt the survivor attitude.
5. Get physical (i.e. exercise).
6. Do not be a "Lone Ranger."
7. Seek support people.
8. Join a support group.
9. Limit your conversations with those who do not understand grief.
10. Be patient with yourself.

In the midst of hard grief made easier by appropriation of Parachin's suggestions, there are things that can complicate the grief process. Wilken and Powell (1993) identify several factors that make male grief more difficult. Once again, these can be applicable to women as well:

- when "strong men" (and women) get lonely
- when pressures of running a household intensify (especially with young or special needs children)
- when couples who have been friends before death distance themselves, either gradually or abruptly
- when men (and women) feel guilty about sex and consider it as "cheating" on dead spouses.

The grief style of one spouse can become a major irritant to the other spouse: for example, when a mother assumes a father is not grieving because he is not emotional; or when the other assumes a partner's grief to be excessive. Some of the variations between the styles of grief can manifest themselves in the following ways (Staudacher, 1991, p. 131):

- differing views on intimacy and sexual desires
- differing views about having other children (particularly if one wants to replace the lost child immediately)
- differing views about methods of raising the surviving child or children (e.g. a hyper-protective mother)
- differing reactions to the other spouse's presence, activities, beliefs, grief.

This chapter has explored the complex nature of grief for men and women. They can grieve differently, but those differences are more related to styles and individual personalities than gender. Grief lingers and does not go away. What can pastoral care givers and others do to support the long pilgrimage of grief? Martin and Doka suggest ten items (1996, pp. 168–169) for care givers to consider. Additional things for consideration will supplement their list:

1. Provide the griever with basic support and comfort.
2. Explore the griever's cognitive responses to death.
3. Reassure the griever that crying and temporary losses of emotional control are normal responses to losing a loved one.
4. Acknowledge all of the griever's affective emotions, but do not insist that he or she cry.
5. Respect the griever's need to withdraw or the need for private space.
6. Encourage constructive venting of hostility, anger, and aggression.
7. When appropriate, assist the griever in recovering emotional self-control.

8. Facilitate a return to useful and meaningful activities previously enjoyed by the griever.
9. Be alert to self-destructive behaviors, especially alcohol and drug use or risk-taking behaviors such as speeding.
10. Gently encourage the griever to seek professional help.

Additional considerations:

1. Do not assume males are not grieving, even if they say they are not grieving.
2. Encourage grievers to do the "hard time" rather than "lite" grief.
3. Listen all of the way to the end of sentences.
4. Acknowledge the spiritual questions.
5. Give grievers permission to be angry at God.
6. Emphasize choices rather than decisions.
7. Give people permission to grieve thoroughly.
8. Help people recognize their own individual style for grief and utilize their strengths.

Finally, the goal of pastoral care with adults, male and female, is the same as the goals for other groups: provide a safe place for people to struggle with and express their feelings about a significant loss and to learn more about the journey called grief. In the book *Beyond Widowhood*, Robert Digiulio has sound advice for adult grievers living in a hectic, fast-paced world:

> *"Give yourself time to move through grief at your own pace and in your own individual way."*
>
> *Robert Digiulio (1989)*

8

Living With Suicide: A Grief Like No Other

"The act or an instance of taking one's own life voluntarily and intentionally..." is the definition of suicide according to *Webster's Seventh New Collegiate Dictionary.* "To kill oneself," though, is a more succinct, matter-of-fact definition. It is simple. However, nothing else about death from suicide is simple, not even the "Why?" Although, theoretically at least, Dr. Max Malikow, a psychotherapist specializing in the treatment of depression and suicide, does have an answer to the "why." He states *"suicide is an act driven by rage (not anger), aloneness (not loneliness), and despair (not depression)"* (1999, p. 44). Determining which of these is the key influence of a given suicide, though, is difficult to assess because everything about death from suicide is far more complex than death by another means, a fact reflected in the words of Kay Redfield Jamison:

> *"Suicide is a death like no other, and those who are left behind to struggle with it must confront a pain like no other ... they are left to the silence of others, who are horrified, embarrassed, or unable to cobble together a note of condolence, an embrace, or a comment ..."*
>
> Kay Redfield Jamison (1999, p. 292)

Furthermore, suicide is not uncommon. According to a January, 1998 report from the Centers for Disease Control and Prevention (CDC), more people in this country die from suicide than from homicide (the same is true today in 2006); over 60% of suicide deaths are not firearm-related. On an average day, 86 people die from suicide, and an estimated 1,900 adults attempt suicide. The CDC report stated that in 1995 suicide took the lives of 31,284 Americans (11.1 people per 100,000 population). Shockingly, Caucasians account for almost 90% of all suicides, and an overwhelming majority of that number are males.

Based upon these statistics, suicide is a major cause of death in the United States. Yet, greater problems exist for the survivors of suicide. According to Mary Pat McMahon, vice-chair for the New England affiliate of the American Foundation for Suicide Prevention (AFSP), the stigma and *"the isolation of being a 'suicide family' underlies the enormous power of this death"* (2000, p. 10). Peggy Farrell, chair of the New Jersey Chapter of the AFSP, relates that this "suicide family" (i.e. people intimately associated with suicide) is estimated to include six persons (1997, p. 35). Therefore, over 200,000 people (31,000 plus suicide victims and survivors) are affected annually in this country because of suicide.

Interestingly, suicide victims are not exclusively those in the mid-years of life. According to a 2005 report of the National Institute for Mental Health, 16.4% of all suicides in 1996 occurred in the lives of people under 25 years of age. This percentage is steadily and staggeringly on the rise. From 1952 to 1995 suicide incidences among adolescents and young adults tripled. Furthermore, from 1980 to 1995, the suicide rate of individuals between the ages of 15 and 19 increased by 23%, and between the ages of 10 and 14 the increase was 112%.

Mary Stimming, citing the CDC findings, states that suicide is the second leading cause of death among college students and the third among teenagers. In 1996, more teenagers and young adults died from suicide than from cancer, heart disease, AIDS, birth defects, stroke, pneumonia, influenza, and chronic lung disease combined (2000, p. 272).

Without question, adolescent and young adult suicide must be taken more seriously. Howard Schubiner relates that for every teenager who commits suicide, 50 or more will make the attempt (1991, p. 51). Moreover, Husain (1990) reports that female young people demonstrate more suicidal gestures and attempts, but young males actually complete more suicides. According to Goodwin and Brown, there are six factors responsible for increased suicide in young people (1989):

1. substance abuse
2. mental illness
3. impulsive, aggressive, and antisocial behavior
4. family influences, including a history of violence and disruption in the family unit
5. severe stress in school or social life
6. rapid sociological change.

The alarmingly high rate of suicide among young people must come down. However, in the face of these six risk factors, how can this happen? Alertness of family, friends, and pastoral care givers to the possibility of suicide is the key.

According to the *Facts for Families: Teen Suicide* article from the American Academy of Child and Adolescent Psychiatry (AACAP), people should be concerned when they notice any of the following 'red flags':

- change in eating and sleeping habits
- withdrawal from friends, family, and regular activities
- violent actions, rebellious behavior, or running away
- drug and alcohol use
- unusual neglect of personal appearance
- marked personality change
- persistent boredom, difficulty concentrating, or a decline in the quality of schoolwork
- frequent complaints about physical symptoms, often related to emotions, such as stomach aches, headaches, fatigue, etc.
- loss of interest in pleasurable activities
- not tolerating praise or rewards.

Furthermore, if any of these attitudes, conversations, or actions follow losses (real or perceived), Schubiner says that such young people should be considered high risks for suicide (1991, p. 51).

Now, we turn our attention to the opposite end of the age spectrum: Suicide among the elderly. According to the January, 1998 CDC report, suicide rates increase with age and are highest among Americans of 65 years of age and older. Of the elderly population, divorced and widowed men showed the highest suicide rates. Men accounted for 82% of this age group in 1995, and the numbers increased

15% during the previous 15-year period (1980—34.8 per 100,000; 1995—39.9 per 100,000). Similarly, during this same 15-year period, the largest increases in suicide rates occurred among those individuals from 80 to 84 years of age. The rate for men in this group increased 19%.

However, risk factors for suicide among the elderly differ from those among the young. For example, older persons at risk for suicide exhibit or have the following characteristics:

- higher prevalence of alcohol abuse
- greater incidents of extreme depression
- social isolation
- greater use of highly lethal methods (e.g. firearms were the most common method of suicide used by both men [74%] and women [31%])
- more physical illnesses of a chronic nature.

Although youth suicide has captured much attention, studies have shown that suicide rates among older Americans are higher and merit closer scrutiny. Probably, one factor influencing the high number of suicides among the elderly is the greater incidence of terminal illnesses.

In an article entitled "Suicide and Terminal Illness," Peter M. Marzuk (1994) states that many self-inflicted deaths among terminally ill patients are never classified as suicides. Therefore, it is difficult to ascertain accurate numbers. However, Marzuk reported that studies show there is a suicide risk among people with cancer, AIDS, and Huntington's chorea. Now, that is not to say that people with other diseases are not at risk; these were the only three cited in the article. Marzuk continues that the predominant mechanism for suicide of the terminally ill is overdose with medications, many of them physician-prescribed. Furthermore, as with other forms of suicide, there are identifiable risk factors for suicide with terminally ill patients (1994, pp. 497–505):

- altered mental state—depression, anxiety, psychosis, and delirium
- hopelessness
- pain and deterioration
- social isolation
- dependency on others
- moving away from home
- financial insolvency.

Several of these risk factors are characteristic of the general population of the elderly. However, suicide of the terminally ill is not exclusive to the elderly. This is especially true of suicide victims who had AIDS. Finally, is suicide of the terminally ill a major problem in this country? It is not. Most people with terminal illnesses do not complete suicide.

Not only are those previously mentioned people groups within the general population at risk for suicide, but vocational groups as well. In an article entitled "Suicide in Law Enforcement: It's Personal," NYPD Lieutenant Robert Kippel (2000) talked about the suicide of three colleagues in December, 1999. His story highlighted risk factors that are not unique to law enforcement but other vocations as well (e.g. firefighters, military personnel).

- Long hours of duty, which prevent officers from spending quality time, or very much time, with their families, can cause personal lives to be precarious. There is the constant threat of separation or divorce.
- Anticipation of retirement is a time of heightened anxiety for police officers. Returning to civilian life is difficult. One feels isolated from camaraderie, powerless, invalidated, all of which contribute to a sense of hopelessness and depression.

Kippel goes on to say that many of the suicides in law enforcement happen at night. Like an illness, other problems appear to be worse when it is dark. When people work extended shifts through long, lonely nights and are not with families or asleep, but awake and often not busy, the mind is at work and the problems embellish. Kippel offers sound advice by suggesting to colleagues that they find a way to *"make it until dawn."* Things will most likely look different in the morning. And somehow they generally do (2000, pp. 11–12). With respect to a person's overall perspective on life, Morrie Schwartz has this to say:

> *"You have to find what's good and true and beautiful in your life as it is now."*
> *Morrie Schwartz (in Albom, 1997, p. 120)*

In the previous pages, we have reviewed statistics highlighting the fact that suicide is a serious public health problem. Among the national mortality averages for the United States, suicide ranks eighth overall. We have also identified people and vocational groups at risk and cited contributing factors for suicide within those groups of which people should be aware. We now turn our attention to the larger number of people affected by suicide: the survivors—family members, friends, coworkers, members of a faith community.

Any death is devastating to surviving loved ones, but death by suicide enlarges and complicates an already emotionally heightened and grief-filled time. Mary Pat McMahon, a mother whose 23-year-old son completed suicide, has this to say about the realities of suicide for victims and survivors:

> *"It is never simple: unforgivable, shameful, stigmatizing, tragic, a release from pain, shocking, mysterious, a way out, a mistake, devastating. These are but some of the things that are the truth about suicide. Those of us who are survivors have been so violated that our souls and spirits are altered forever."*
> *Mary Pat McMahon (2000, p. 10)*

In an article entitled "Death by Any Other Name," Tamina Toray (2000) relates the haunting experience of her father's suicide and its effect on her as an 11-year-old child. The shock of the death of her father rendered her mother unable to be there for Toray. Even as an adult, Toray says that the impact of her mother's absence on her grief is still hard to assess. Furthermore, the return to school was a nightmare. No adult there spoke a word about her father's death. It was quite obvious that discomfort was experienced by teachers and peers. She states that she was emotionally isolated by her peers and viewed as an anomaly by her teachers.

> *"The need for adult support intervention was acute and yet none was available."*
> *Tamina Toray (2000)*

How piercing are Toray's words "... none was available"—at least not immediately and not from people you would expect, like school personnel, family, or faith congregation. Help did come, though, six months after her father's death, in the person of a summer camp counselor. Toray testifies that a relationship with a caring adult can make a dramatic difference in the life of a child who has endured a great hardship (2000, pp. 4–5). In addition to the truths of suicide shared by McMahon, Toray provides others: *isolation, silence, lack of support*. She also has this to say about loss from suicide:

> *"Death by suicide differs from all other deaths in that such a death narrows the lens from which the deceased person's life is viewed. My father became the 'suicide' ... His life became the mode of his death, leaving my memories to this day focused on a moment of horror and violence not on a lifetime of diverse events. Healthy grieving involves a savoring of a variety of memories of the deceased; yet, a suicide reduces those memories to one moment of terror increasing the likelihood of complicated grief."*
>
> *Tamina Toray (2000)*

How poignant are her words. "Death by suicide is unthinkable," so many people say. "What a shameful and tragic end to a life." "How could anyone do such a thing?" Attitudes about suicide which produce comments like these, silence, alienation, etc., have greatly enhanced the shame and stigma associated with suicide. Moreover, similar statements have driven suicide families underground. Consequently, they do not get the needed help for reconciliation with the loss, and grief can become compounded. According to Peggy Farrell (1997), the basis for such negative perception of suicide victims results from a misunderstanding about the primary underlying factor that causes suicide.

For centuries, people believed suicide was a moral issue. Some religious traditions deemed it a sin, even unpardonable. Family members were often blamed for the person's death. It was believed that other people did something so horrific that the person was driven to suicide. This attitude prompted communities to force suicide families to move away. In the Middle Ages in Great Britain, families were expected to pay a fine to the crown if one of their members committed suicide.

Today, though, it is widely known that suicide is most often the result of a major mental illness or breakdown and biochemical in nature. If you will refer back to the risk factors associated with various people and occupational groups, the vast majority had nothing to do with moral concerns, but things precipitated by emotional issues. Even so, the mark of shame still exists for suicide because of the stigma associated with mental illness. Nevertheless, bereavement from suicide is, and perhaps always will be, a grief like no other kind. While it is true that suicide grievers exhibit similar emotions and behaviors to those of grievers of death by other means, there are grief issues more clearly associated with death by suicide. In an article entitled "Is Suicide Bereavement Different?" John R. Jordan provides a list of suicide grief issues encountered by the victims' survivors (2000, pp. 2–3):

- heightened feelings of responsibility for the death (this is experienced to some degree in other deaths as well, for example, child/teen death, line-of-duty death)
- rejection by the deceased
- greater questions about the deceased's motivation for not living
- intensified feelings that they (survivors) should have prevented the death

- higher frequency of hiding the cause of death from other people
- strong tendencies toward feelings of shame and embarrassment about the death
- more difficulty in making meaning or sense of the death
- more feelings of anger toward the deceased for the perceived abandonment in the death
- expectation that others will judge them more harshly as mourners of a suicide because studies indicate that society still holds negative feelings toward suicide
- expenditure of much more psychological energy attempting to comprehend the reason(s) for the death
- increased risk of suicide among suicide mourners

All of these and, most certainly, more issues encountered by survivor families are what led Mary Pat McMahon to describe the aftermath of her son Matt's suicide:

> *"We are never, ever the same after losing a loved one to suicide."*
> Mary Pat McMahon (2000, p. 10)

As true as that statement is, life can be meaningful again for suicide survivors' families. John Jordan suggests that trained care givers can be important resources and referral agents for support of suicide survivors if they educate themselves about the causes of suicide and the unique aspects of suicide grief (2000, p. 3). One very important element of pastoral care with survivor families is the articulation of effective listening. Max Malikow provides some helpful "Do's" and "Don'ts" (1999, pp. 42, 44):

Do's

- Do be an active listener by not only observing body language, but by asking questions for clarification. Practice basic attending skills such as the minimal encourage, paraphrase, reflection of feeling, and summarization to reassure the grievers that they are heard and understood.
- Do listen for the five most common concerns of suicide survivors:
  1. need to know why
  2. guilt
  3. anger
  4. finding someone to blame
  5. fear that they, too, are capable of suicide.
- Do seize the opportunity to make a referral because these five common concerns indicate one is in order.

In response to Malikow's final "Do" about making a referral, we want to mention two sources for referrals: homogeneous support groups and friends of survivor families. Concerning the former, John R. Jordan recounts:

> *"Most (suicide) survivors seem to feel that their experience is different from those with other types of losses, and often believe that other survivors are the people most likely to understand them without judging the suicide or their grief."*
> John R. Jordan (2000, p. 3)

There are also other distinct benefits of a homogeneous support group:

- shelter against isolation and despair (Mary Pat McMahon)
- commonality of shared experiences facilitates healing (Peggy Farrell)

- more rapid coherence of grievers because of exclusivity of group (John R. Jordan)
- highlights the importance of community as a key element in helping to bring about a re-bonding with self and the world that has been shattered by the death (Mary Pat McMahon).

With respect to the latter, Victor M. Parachin enumerates several ways that friends can render aid in those deep, dark hours of despair following the suicide of a loved one (1998a, pp. 6, 8):

- Friends show up and provide hospitality, all the while affirming life by talking, crying, hugging, laughing.
- Friends show up with open arms and do not say a word. The warm embraces and tears powerfully communicate genuine caring.
- Friends help in practical ways (e.g. providing food for physical nourishment, plants and fresh flowers which symbolize life and hope, finances to help with unplanned expenses).
- Friends attend the funeral or memorial service as a symbol and reminder to the survivor family that they are loved.
- Friends stand with the survivors for the long haul to help in the rebuilding of lives.
- Friends encourage survivors to turn the tragedy of their loss into something positive (e.g. starting a support group for suicide survivors in the community).
- Friends do not allow survivors to withdraw from life.

Don'ts

- Do not answer questions that have not been asked.
- Do not take exclamations like "Why did this have to happen?" as questions requiring an answer.
- Do not pointedly answer questions that are:
  - theological—"How does God judge a suicide?"
  - psychological— "Why do people commit suicide?"
  - medical— "Could (a particular drug) have caused this?"
- As opposed to giving specific answers to questions like these, it is better for the care giver to respond with other questions as a way to facilitate self-discovery on the part of the griever. For example, in response to the theological question mentioned above, the dialogue could look something like, "How do you think God judges suicide? ... Why do you think that? ... Have you considered this possibility? ..." etc. The same principle follows for other questions as well: "Why do you think people complete suicide? ..."

Before concluding this chapter with some final thoughts for pastoral care givers, we want to discuss how to talk to children as members of a surviving family. In an article entitled "Suicide: How Can We Talk to the Children?" (2000), Linda Goldman says:

> *"Our inability to discuss the topic of suicide openly with children can create an atmosphere of fear, isolation and loneliness that can be far more devastating than the death of a loved one."*
>
> *Linda Goldman (2000, p. 6)*

It is normal and healthy for children to grieve the loss of a family member or friend. Enabling them to experience the grief process without creating additional barriers prompted by the typical adult perception is the challenge of grief care givers. Furthermore, it is very important to reinforce the concept that the child was not the cause of the death. Goldman states that openness about suicide can be achieved in two ways (2000, pp. 6–7):

1. Stress the principle that we always need to separate the person who died from the way that person died to truly grieve the person's death. (That is excellent advice for adults as well.)

   "A person's life was more than the moment of death."

   Nancy Crump

2. Define suicide and certain things typically associated with it to children in simple, direct, age-appropriate language that eliminates judgment.
   - Suicide—The act of killing yourself so that your body won't work anymore. People may do this when they feel there is no other way they can think of to solve their problems. However, there is always another way.
   - Death—Death is when a person's body stops working.
   - Grief—The natural feelings we feel after someone close to us has died. These feelings can be sadness, anger, fear, guilt, depression.
   - Guilt—A feeling that makes us think we are the cause of something or that we may have done something wrong.
   - Depression—Extreme feelings of sadness and hopelessness that last a long time.

Definitions are all well and good, but how does a parent or other adult actually dialogue with a child about the suicide of a loved one? Goldman shares some practical suggestions to guide discussion (2000, pp. 7, 9):

- **Define suicide** as when someone chooses to make his or her own body stop working.
- **Relate age-appropriate facts and explanations.** "One day Mommy took too many pills. She had been having a lot of problems lately. Mom acted really sad and would sometimes do strange things."
- **Retell good memories.** "Mommy loved you. When she wasn't feeling bad she loved being with you. Remember the fun time we had together ...''
- **Dispel myths of suicide.** "We do not know all the reasons why people do this. Just because Mommy did not want her body to work anymore does not mean that the same thing will happen to me or even you. Daddy will not leave you." (Be careful making promises to a child.)
- **Model feelings and thoughts.** "I wish Mommy would not have left us. I wished she would have tried harder. I'm sort of mad at Mommy for leaving us because I miss her so much. I also still love her very much."
- **Provide alternatives.** "Mommy was wrong to do this. She felt that making her body stop working was the only way. I don't know what the right answer was, but this wasn't it. There was another way."
- **Use third person language** because it is less threatening to children, and it enables them to open up more easily. "Some people say that making your body stop working is ...''

Even after having that difficult talk of explaining what happened, the task of caring for children in grief is just beginning. Children can and do experience the same emotions as adults. They can feel ashamed of the death, guilty over the death, angry at the death, and depressed about the death. Children can also have suicidal thoughts, as can adults. The problem arises in perceiving what these feelings are because young children may not have the language or emotional maturity to express them. Therefore, silence and differing behaviors emerge that are tell-tale signs of complexity in processing the tragedy. Goldman provides a list of activities and feelings of which adults need to be aware as indicators of problems (2000, p. 9):

- Outbursts of aggressiveness or withdrawal.
- Extreme feelings of unworthiness or powerlessness.
- Conflicted relationship with the deceased.
- Extreme guilt and over-responsibility about the deceased.
- Hyperactivity, impulsivity, and inability to concentrate.
- Withdrawal from social activities.
- Giving away possessions and planning their own funerals.
- Nightmares.

(All of these can be indicators of problems in grievers of any age.)

- Bedwetting.
- Poor grades in school.
- Withdrawal from school.

(Any of these symptoms can be found in children experiencing death by other means as well.)

Noticing any of these behaviors or expressions of feelings can be an indicator that the child is at risk: depressed at best or possibly suicidal. Care givers need to be vigilant in screening at-risk children, beginning in elementary school, says Goldman. There are two questions to which she says depressed children respond consistently in a positive manner:

1. Do you feel sad all of the time?
2. Do you feel hopeless all of the time?

Furthermore, Goldman suggests that care givers use a simple at-risk screening tool with young children. Ask them to write or draw their responses to the following questions:

- What makes you the angriest?
- What makes you very sad?
- What do you wish for the most?
- What scares you the most?

With respect to the last of those questions, it is quite common for children to fear the death of a surviving parent. This fear is heightened when the death of one parent is through suicide (Toray, 2000, p. 5).

Lastly, we want to offer some approaches for suicide ministry to pastoral care givers, a primary one being patience—a fact highlighted by Mary Pat McMahon:

"We need to be heard for a longer time than other bereaved."
Mary Pat McMahon (2000, p. 10)

McMahon's words underscore those of William Shakespeare (cited by Malikow, 1999):

> *"How poor are the impatient. For what wound did ever heal but by degrees?"*
> *William Shakespeare (cited by Malikow, 1999, p. 44)*

Pastoral care givers also need to keep in mind these things in ministry to suicide victims' survivors:

- Do not compare other losses through death unless those other losses were by suicide (McMahon).
- Attempt to assure survivor families of God's companionship and faithfulness in their days of despair (Stimming).
- Professional support is necessary for a healthy recovery. If you intend to have an effective ministry with suicide families, educate yourself about this very different kind of grief.
- Peer support is also necessary for a healthy recovery. Make referrals to appropriate support groups.
- "Ask us 'how we are' and risk the answer" (McMahon).
- Love the survivor families unconditionally.

> *"Sensitivity to and compassion for suicide survivor families are the key elements in effective pastoral care."*
>
> *SLJ*

9

Stages of Grief: Fact or Fiction?

Until recent times, grievers experienced no time pressure or sense of urgency to get over the death of a dear loved one. "Take as long as you need" was the common guidance given by grief supporters. President Dwight David Eisenhower wrote to a grieving father 25 years after the death of his own son, Ikky, telling him not to expect to ever get over a daughter's death. In his book *Eisenhower* (1999), Geoffrey Perret noted that the leader of the free world "... *never stopped grieving over Ikky, and never would.*"

> *"Grief is a complex life experience, replete with ambiguity and fraught with great difficulty."*
>
> *SLJ*

Few would doubt the truth of that statement. However, since the advent of the 1960s and the space age inaugurated by the young, charismatic President John Fitzgerald Kennedy, there became little tolerance for complexity, ambiguity, and difficulty. The new generation lauded simplicity, clarity, possibility, and such were to be achieved through forward thinking and innovation. Even grief therapy was not immune to societal changes and would itself undergo quite a transformation.

During that decade, Elisabeth Kubler-Ross' work (1969) with dying patients began that transformation and got people talking about dying, death, and grief. The five-stage model for dealing with grief during the dying process she postulated has, unfortunately, been superimposed by counselors and laity for grief associated with death. Her model is as follows:

Denial → Anger → Bargaining → Depression → Acceptance

Kubler-Ross' method is the only model for "doing grief" that some pastoral care givers and healthcare professionals know and use. A major reason for this is that her model is the one predominately taught in graduate programs in medicine and nursing. This is the conclusion reached by Downe-Wambolt and Tamlyn who recorded the findings of their research in a 1997 article in *Death Studies* entitled "An International Survey of Death Education Trends in Faculties of Nursing and Medicine." This work was preceded by a piece authored by Coolican, Stark, Doka, and Corr on "Education about Death, Dying, and Bereavement in Nursing Programs," which was featured in a 1994 edition of *Nurse Educator*. Of course, there are other studies of a similar nature by grief specialists who draw the same conclusions concerning the prevalence and dominance of Kubler-Ross' five-stage model.

> *"Kubler-Ross was an early leader and an important publicist for efforts to understand coping and dying."*
>
> *Charles A. Corr (1993, p. 81)*

Even though Corr is not an avid devotee of Kubler-Ross, he does see a tremendous value in her work and recognizes that she did alert pastoral and mental health care givers to three realities among grievers.

1. Grievers often have unfinished business that needs to be addressed to facilitate reconciliation with the death.
2. Care givers cannot effectively offer help without listening deliberately to those who are bereaved in order to help them identify their needs.
3. Care givers need to learn from the grieving in order to know themselves better and, thus, to offer better pastoral care.

> *"Although we all benefited from the work of Kubler-Ross, we cannot simply lean upon her work for the rest of time ... we must look within ourselves to go beyond the inadequacies of the stage-based model for coping with dying that Kubler-Ross set forth so many years ago."*
>
> *Charles A. Corr (1993, p. 81)*

The intent of this section is not to delve deeply into a discussion of the Kubler-Ross model of grief. Her work was important but is now dated. Our goal is two-fold:

1. to introduce other stage models of grief for consideration; and
2. to call attention to limitations of and objections to stage models for healthy grieving as outlined by several grief specialists.

But first: why were and are such stage systems so popular?

> *"Simple step-by-step models of this kind are appealing for their clarity, a factor that has contributed to their widespread appeal among both professionals and lay persons striving to understand the complexities of loss."*
>
> *Robert A. Neimeyer (1998, p. 84)*

Significant in Neimeyer's assessment are the words "simple" and "complexities." We call your attention to the introduction to this chapter in which we suggested that the "new generation" sought to replace complexity with simplicity.

Wayne Oates

Oates suggested grief is expressed in six stages, which may or may not be "telescoped" into each other (*see* Wayne Oates, *Anxiety in Christian Experience*):

1. Shocking blow of loss-in-itself.
2. Numbing effect of the shock.
3. Struggle between fantasy and reality.
4. Break-through of a flood of grief.
5. Selective memory and stabbing pain.
6. Acceptance of loss and reaffirmation of life itself.

David Switzer

Switzer recognized four common phases of grief (*see* David Switzer, *The Minister as Crisis Counselor*, 1974, pp. 149–152):

1. Feeling of numbness and denial.

2. Yearning for and preoccupation with thoughts of the deceased person.
3. Disorganization and despair.
4. Reorganization of behavior.

John Bowlby

Bowlby argued that the four stages (phases) are not clear cut and may flip-flop, intertwine, but are generally not in a straight line of progression (*see* John Bowlby, 1980):

1. *Numbing* lasting from a few hours to a week, but may be interrupted by outbursts of extremely intense distress.
2. *Yearning and searching for the lost individual* lasting for months and sometimes even for years.
3. *Disorganization and despair* emerge when the reality of death cannot be denied, in which many emotions are now evident, especially depression and guilt.
4. *Reorganization* of a greater or lesser degree as the bereaved adjusts to the loss.

Carl Nighswonger

Nighswonger, a chaplain who worked with Kubler-Ross, saw the care giver's task as helping dying persons experience their own grief. He viewed the process as a series of dramas (*see* Carl Nighswonger, "Ministry to the Dying as a Learning Encounter," 1972):

1. Drama of shock: Denial versus panic.
2. Drama of emotion: Catharsis versus depression.
3. Drama of negotiation: Bargaining versus selling out.
4. Drama of cognition: Realistic hope versus despair.
5. Drama of commitment: Acceptance versus resignation.
6. Drama of completion: Fulfillment versus forlornness.

Erich Lindemann

Lindemann followed, for many years, the families of the several hundred casualties who died in the November 28, 1942 Coconut Grove Night Club fire in Boston, Massachusetts. He identified five stages of acute grief by looking at reactions of grieving persons (*see* Erich Lindemann, *Beyond Grief: Studies in Crisis Intervention*, 1986, pp. 59–78):

1. Somatic distress.
2. Preoccupation with the image of the deceased.
3. Guilt.
4. Hostile reactions.
5. Loss of patterns of conduct.

Donald Capps

Capps designed a process of grief stages based on spirituality. His guiding principle is that working through painful feelings is an indispensable part of comfort; blocked feelings delay or block comfort (*see* Donald Capps, 2003).

1. Address to God.
2. Complaint—venting negative feelings.
3. Confession of trust—sense of being "upheld" and able to cope.
4. Petition of specific needs.
5. Words of assurance.
6. Vow to praise.

J. Thomas Meigs

Meigs suggested that the inevitable question for the bereaved is, *"How do I make the necessary shifts from living with the dead to living without the dead?"* He stated that certain things need to be done in order for one to move ahead (J Thomas Meigs, 1984).

1. Deal with the emotions of grief.
2. Put the relationship with the deceased in perspective as an important part of the past; grief elicits strong loyalty to the past. If one keeps a "shrine," there will be difficulty completing bereavement.
3. Redefine roles and relationships in light of the significant loss, rather than living for the dead.
4. Affirm the right to live in the present and the future without the deceased. Be open to possibilities of new relationships, new friendships, new meanings in life and a new self-identity and appreciation of self.

These are only a sample of the many theories of grief that have evolved since the work of Kubler-Ross. One striking feature of these theories is the similarities among them. Differences are usually semantic in nature.

Robert J. Kastenbaum summarizes limitations of and objections to stage theories (1986):

• The existence of these stages has not been demonstrated by empirical research.
• No evidence demonstrates that grievers actually move from stage one to stage five in a clear, linear progression.
• The limitations of the methods that led to the development of the theory have not been acknowledged.
• The line is blurred between description and prescription.
• The totality of a person's life (e.g. previous losses) is neglected in favor of the supposed stages.
• Resources, pressures and characteristics of the immediate environment, which cannot be ignored, are not considered.

While bereavement is a universal phenomenon, individuals experience grief uniquely. Because of this fact, stage theory opponents suggest that the identification of stages as "normal" grief impedes a person's freedom to grieve uniquely and thoroughly. Observe this liberating insight by Charles A. Corr:

> "No one has to [grieve] in any particular way. To insist that individuals must cope... in what others regard as the 'right' or 'correct' way is simply to impose the additional burdens of an external agenda upon vulnerable persons."
>
> Charles A. Corr (1993)

Increasingly, thanatologists (professionals who study death and bereavement) and professional pastoral care givers recognize, in their opinions, the inadequacy of stage models of grief. In fact, Kubler-Ross' five stages model has been soundly rejected by several grief scholars (Feigenberg, 1980; Kastenbaum, 1998; Pattison, 1977; Shneidman, 1980/1995; and Weisman, 1972; and more recently by Neimeyer, 1998). The following statement reflects the reticence of many scholars and practitioners to stage models of grief.

> "Schematic stages— denial, anger, bargaining, depression, acceptance—are at best approximations, and at worst, obstacles to individualization."
>
> A. D. Weisman (1972, p. 121)

Furthermore, E. M. Pattison insists that stages "may oversimplify coping processes and suppress individuality in coping" (1977, cited in Corr, Doka and Kastenbaum, 1999, p. 246) and thus be counterproductive and impede grief work. After having laid the groundwork for objections to stage thinking, we will now point out several notable, arguably important concerns.

Stages Reduce the Mystery of Death

Death is a mystery; always has been, always will be. Who lives and who dies is a mystery, even in this age of medical sophistication with its dazzling technology. Who, though, has the time to wrestle with mystery in this hustle-bustle world? Admittedly, there are few who have or take the time. Help, though, is now available to address that problem in stage theories which reduce the mystery of death to a quantitative experience. Thus, grievers are encouraged to "stay busy," to keep up the pace in this "fast-lane" society, and get over death and "move on" rather than fully embracing the journey towards reconciliation with the loss. However, if one does not take (make) time to ponder and grapple with the mystery of death, the grief is not reconciled and then it becomes delayed grief, at best.

Stages Are Linear Rather Than Cyclical

Stage theory advocates generally assume that people must complete the stages in something of a linear, orderly, and predictable fashion. Those attempting to cope with bereavement are forced into what Corr, Nabe, and Corr describe in *Death and Dying: Life and Living* (1997, p. 154) as "a pre-established framework that reduces their individuality to little more than an instance of one of five categories ... in a schematic process." The reality is that grievers get caught in the emotional and spiritual cul-de-sacs of denial, anger, bargaining, depression, and acceptance.

Many people understand the stage theories as resembling a check-off list. "Let's see, I've done the denial and the anger. Now, on to the bargaining." For others, stage thinking is similar to school. You begin with *denial* (first grade) and keep on going until you reach *acceptance*, after which you graduate with a diploma. I (HIS) often teach that there is a sixth stage: over-it-land. As generally taught, the stage theory is focused on and emphasizes a desired end result—getting over the death. The reality of grief, though, is that grief is *doing*, and such may well be captured in this phrase: "Three steps forward and two backward, or, in some cases, two steps forward and three backward."

> *"Accept what you are able to do and what you are not able to do."*

Stages Are Scientifically Questionable

Robert Neimeyer in *Lessons of Loss* (1998) states: *"the paucity of empirical evidence to support stage models as well as my clinical observations and experience with loss have led me to reject many of the implicit assumptions of traditional grief theories leading to 'an end state of recovery.'"* He adds, *"the particular form of response and the sequences and duration of the emotional reactions to loss vary greatly among individuals"* (p. 84).

Simply because something is succinct and straightforward, can be easily communicated and embraced by many practitioners, does not make it the unquestionable standard.

Grievers need to be encouraged to live out their grief without having to conform to a model, which is suspect at best. Furthermore, pastoral care givers are called to be witnesses to each unique pilgrimage in which there are no easy answers. The truth is that, in many cases, there well may not be any answers. The relevance of that last statement is poignantly reflected in the words of a grieving mother whose son died in the terrorist attack which caused the crash of Pan Am Flight 103 (cited in Worden, 1991):

> *"It is not how to find an answer, but how to live without one."*
>
> *Cited in Worden (1991, p. 16)*

Stages Focus on Emotional Responses Rather Than "Meaning-Making"

Pastoral care givers who exclusively, or at least primarily, use stage-based models of grief in working with the bereaved typically evaluate progress (or lack thereof) through the stages upon an individual's emotional responses. Those who meet the expectations are praised. Conversely, those who deviate from the pattern of expectant normalcy might be labeled abnormal or pathological and referred to a mental health professional (Neimeyer, 1998). However, pastoral care is not about evaluating emotional responses. On the contrary, responsible care giving is about assisting grievers to search for and to make meaning out of their experiences with death, even to consider grief in the same way as Doug Manning:

> *"Grief is not an enemy—it is a friend. It is a natural process of walking through hurt and growing because of the walk. Let it happen."*
>
> *Doug Manning (1979, p. 61)*

In essence, pastoral care is about offering hospitality to grievers, most commonly through listening. Why should we listen to grievers as opposed to offering them counsel? Thomas Oden tells us: *"Listen carefully to the unparalleled expertise"* (1983, p. 302). Whose expertise is it? Obviously, it is that of the griever. He or she has much to share and needs to do so. The one who takes the time to be an interested, compassionate listener can help to bring about meaning.

Stages Focus on the Chief Mourner Rather Than on Others Impacted by the Death

Unfortunately, the "pure" practitioners of stage theories, by focusing exclusively on the small circle of chief mourners, overlook the extended family, social net-works, and the larger community affected by a death. Commonly, friends—even best friends—are expected to put their grief on the "back burner" in order to "be there for the family." Robert Neimeyer contends that *"loss can only be understood in a broader social context"* (1998, p. 7).

We have presented the stage-based theory of Elisabeth Kubler-Ross as well as modifications of that theory by other grief specialists. We have noted objections to the stages model put forth by still other grief specialists. *To stage or not to stage is the question.* Certainly, stages can be a resource in the care giver's repertoire for it is well known that the phases postulated by the stage theory proponents are validated in the lives of grievers. Many do deny the death; get angry; bargain; experience depression; accept the loss. The reality is, though, that the stages do not necessarily happen in any particular order, and some of them may be experienced simul-taneously (or not at all). Kubler-Ross readily admits this (1969, p. 138). Therefore, a pastoral care giver who offers only the stages as the approach to grief ministry and does not listen to the lived-out experience of the griever, is not providing adequate care.

At this point, we want to introduce another more current model postulated by William Worden who defined the grief process in terms of tasks to be accomplished. (*See* William Worden, *Grief Counseling and Grief Therapy*, 2001, 3rd edition.)

1. **To accept reality of loss.**
   When death is sudden and unexpected, this can be an understandable problem; but even when there has been a long terminal illness an air of unreality and numbness usually descends on the family. Attending the funeral, seeing the body in the coffin are all ways in which the bereaved can be helped to accept the reality of the loss.
2. **To work through to the pain of grief.**
   This can be literal physical pain as well as emotional, and is quite the opposite of denial and numbness. It can manifest itself as sleeplessness, loss of appetite, fatigue, helplessness, shock, and excessive use of alcohol, tranquilizers, etc. There may be a whole range of seemingly contradictory feelings: sadness and relief, anger and a sense of emancipation, anxiety and self-reproach. It is a spiritual as well as a psychological truth that the only way to get through pain is to "go through" pain, not try to avoid it. Doing the "hard time" is a helpful way to health.

Unfortunately, many pastoral care leaders miss the "to" in Worden's task. The task is not to work through but to work through *to* the pain.

3. **To adjust to an environment in which the deceased is missing.**
   Worden (1991) says, *"Adjusting to a new environment means different things to different people, depending on what the relationship was with the deceased and the various roles the deceased played. For many widows or widowers it takes a considerable period of time to realize what it is like to live without their husbands or wives. This realization often begins to emerge around three months after the loss and involves coming to terms with living alone, raising children alone, facing an empty house, and managing finances alone ... The survivor usually is not aware of all the roles played by the deceased until after the loss occurs."* And this requires adjustment, in some instances, to multiple environments: home, school, church.

4. **To emotionally relocate and memorialize the deceased.**
   The bereaved are beginning the resolution process of dealing with the loss. "It happened; there is nothing I can do about it; life goes on." Potential difficulties in this task of grief are feelings of guilt about investing energy in something or someone else and/or belief that "I am betraying the memory of my ..." This is often the most difficult grieving task to accomplish, and the gentle encouragement, reassurance, and "permission" can be critical at this time.

We also want you to be aware of another model by Therese Rando called the "6 'R' Processes of Mourning" found in her benchmark book *Treatment of Complicated Mourning* (1993, p. 45).

1. **Recognize the loss**—acknowledge and understand the death.
2. **React to the separation**—experience the pain; feel, identify, accept, and give some form of expression to all the reactions to the loss; and identify and mourn any secondary losses.
3. **Recollect and re-experience the deceased and the relationship**—review and remember realistically; revive and re-experience the feelings.
4. **Relinquish the old attachments to the deceased**—lay aside the old assumptive mindset that the deceased still exists; the world with him or her is over.
5. **Readjust to move adaptively into the new world without forgetting the old**—revise the assumptive world; develop a new relationship with the deceased; adopt new ways of being in the new world without the deceased; and begin forming a new identity for yourself.
6. **Reinvest**—put your energies in new things and establishing relationships with other people in your new identity.

We highly recommend that you consider these models of Worden and Rando as resources to employ in care of the bereaved.

In conclusion, it is important to remember that the goal of pastoral care with the bereaved is to accompany faithfully those who are *forever changed* by the death of a loved one.

And so, we encourage you to consider the stages models and the alternatives suggested by those who see their limitations. Reread this chapter and ask yourself how your pastoral care skills can be more finely tuned by combining the material presented into an approach that is unique to you. There is no correct way to do grief counseling. Each situation you encounter will be different because no two people, even in the same marriage or family, are the same when it comes to grieving.

"Any time someone suggests that you are not grieving correctly, just glance at your thumb: You are unique and so is your grief."

HIS

We must remember that the most important issue in dealing with the bereaved is not our agenda or "system" for dealing with grief. On the contrary, of ultimate concern is the welfare and spiritual wellness of the griever. Any fresh ideas and new insights, which could enhance our ministry with the bereaved, should be welcomed with open arms. We call your attention to the wisdom of Thomas Oden:

"The experienced minister knows that the times of approaching death and bereavement are exceptional opportunities for spiritual growth. Sensitive care is required to nurture them toward their fullest potentiality and not let them become an occasion for stumbling."

Thomas Oden (1983, p. 297)

10

Where is God?

The title of this chapter is not a common question among grievers. However, it is only the beginning of many subsequent similar interrogative or declarative statements.

- "How could a loving God let this happen?"
- "God could have healed my loved one, but He didn't."
- "Nothing makes sense anymore."
- "God, I am angry at you!"
- "I don't think you even care."
- "I am not even sure you exist."
- "Why?"
- "Why now?"
- "Why this?"
- "Why me?"
- "What am I supposed to do now?"

Grievers have questions of ultimate concern, even those who are devoutly religious. Death can and often does invalidate one's belief system, or at least calls it into violent question. It devastates some and tests others' spirituality as indicated by the questions asked. Since pastoral care givers are God's field representatives, they are supposed to have answers to these questions. That is correct, is it not? The reality is that many of the questions asked will not be answerable, but they are normal questions in times of distress, like the death of a loved one. Gerald Sittser, whose mother, wife, and daughter died in an automobile crash, asked many of those normal questions and had these words to say:

> "Loss may call the existence of God into question. Pain seems to conceal him from us, making it hard for us to believe that there could be a God in the midst of our suffering. In our pain we are tempted to reject God, yet for some reason we hesitate to take that course of action. So we ponder and pray. We move toward God, then away from him."
>
> Gerald Sittser (1995, p. 144)

This blinding pain can be physical, emotional, and spiritual. Without question, death does bring with it inescapable questions of a spiritual nature, which paralyze some grievers and energize others. The ones in the latter group can and will ask their questions with the zeal of a seasoned prosecutor. Such barrages of an intense nature can well cause some pastoral care givers to feel most uncomfortable and even defensive, particularly if the exchange is public. What is an appropriate pastoral care response to these questions? One thing is certain; the questioners are not really expecting answers for many of their questions, for they know there are none. In many cases, grievers are simply venting their frustrations and anxieties. Thus, what bereaved individuals need in those times of heightened anguish is someone to listen to what they have to say and be a faithful witness in their struggles to live with unanswerable, taunting questions. They desire someone who will be patient with them and understanding of their "temporary atheism/agnosticism."

"Practice the sacrament of presence: Be there and be actively quiet."

SLJ

Having said that, it is healthy for grievers to be vocal about challenges to their assumptions, spiritual and otherwise. When the bereaved cannot or do not verbalize questions and concerns, they suffer in isolation. In situations where this silence is so thick you could cut it with a knife, a pastoral care giver (or a griever) can stimulate meaningful dialogue by proposing a thought-provoking question: "Are you angry, even angry at God?"

Unfortunately, many people are afraid to express anger at or question God. What they need then is permission from a representative of God that to be angry at God is okay for He fully understands that they do not understand why their loved one died. They also need the affirmation that God will not reject them or pay them back for anger directed at Him. On the contrary, if anything, God moves ever closer in such times in order to provide comfort, love, and assurance that those who are hurt and angry are very special to Him.

Furthermore, God wants people to be honest with Him about their feelings. One moving moment in the movie *Shadowlands* reflects the type of honesty God honors. After seven-year-old Douglas' mother died, he asked his stepfather, C. S. Lewis, *"Do you believe in heaven?"* Lewis replied: *"Yes, I do."* Douglas responded, *"I don't believe in heaven any more."* After a short pause, Lewis said: *"That's okay."* The great Cambridge professor gave the young boy permission to honestly acknowledge his feelings. As a pastoral care giver, you can do the same. Astute care givers will also recognize that such situations are neither the time nor the place for theological instruction to correct, what is, in their opinion, errant statements, or to engage in deep dialogue in response to questions: Reflections, yes; arguments, no. Occasions for theological discussions are better suited for a later time at the initiative of the grievers.

Moreover, there are certain types of death that, according to Robert Neimeyer, *"challenge the adequacy of our most cherished beliefs and taken-for-granted ways of life"* (1998, p. 88). I would qualify Neimeyer's statement by adding "more significantly" before the word "challenge," because virtually all deaths challenge our belief systems. The type of deaths, though, to which he refers are those "out-of-order deaths" (suicide of a mate, tragic drowning of a child, an automobile accident killing a bride and groom, random violence that takes the lives of teens, line-of-duty deaths of public servants, etc.) Some deaths place many grievers on a collision course with their beliefs about God.

Consider the following real-life scenarios. Newlyweds are supposed to grow old together, not die in a car wreck on their honeymoon. Children are supposed to grow up and bury parents, not parents burying children. Fire and police department personnel are supposed to go home following a shift, not die in the line of duty. So, where was God when these things happened? Where was God on an April day in 1999 when two students brutally executed several of their peers and a teacher at Columbine High School in Littleton, Colorado? Where was God on September 11, 2001? Where is God when multiple tragedies of various kinds happen repeatedly on a daily basis around the globe?

Additionally, pastoral care givers themselves are not immune to grief or doubts. C. S. Lewis, author of *A Grief Observed*, was recognized by many to be a theological authority on suffering and pain. However, after the deaths of his close friend, Charles Williams, and his wife, Joy, Lewis confessed: *"I thought I trusted the rope until it mattered to me whether it would bear me. Now it matters, and I find I didn't"* (1961, p. 43). Unfortunately, the apparent meaning of those words is shrouded in philosophical jargon. To put it plainly, Lewis is saying, "I had faith until I needed it, then I didn't." Consigned to the laboratory of grief, the great philosopher/theologian began to re-examine his most cherished beliefs, along with the "answers" he had given others in his lectures, radio broadcasts, and writings.

> *"Grief is an experience that can stretch the limits of one's faith."*
>
> *SLJ*

Finally, for people of diverse religious traditions, death brings about a series of questions:

- questions about the divine
- questions about the afterlife
- questions about hope
- questions about punishment.

As one who administers pastoral care, you will be called upon to walk with the griever step by step, forward and backward, grappling with those difficult, sometimes unanswerable questions. During those journeys, remember this one thing:

> *"It is not so much what you say or do that is important in those moments, but who you are: a nonjudgmental, caring presence."*
>
> *SLJ*

11

Is There Life After Death For Me?

"My life is over."
"How can I go on living?"
"She was my life. What am I going to do without her?
"Life is no longer worth living."

Questions are often asked and statements made by the bereaved about their own lives after the deaths of loved ones. In fact, there does not even have to be a death to elicit such responses. Teenagers talk about life after a relationship is severed. Similarly, divorcees relate sentiments of like kind following the breakup of a marriage. People who lose their jobs and, sometimes, even retirees speak about life subsequent to termination from employment, whether involuntary or voluntary. Of course, those questions and statements about life address the strong possibility that there will be no life, or if there is life, it will have little or no quality.

Over and beyond those times of crisis that cause people to question the very existence of life, human beings are continually constructing their own unique worlds in the attempt to define and comprehend meaning personally and in relationship to others:

- what life means to be *me*
- what life means to be *you*
- what life means to be *us*.

However, death disrupts and makes shambles of people's lives. Many feel like Humpty Dumpty. "My life can never be put back together again." But it can.

The survivor, the one cut loose from the mooring and adrift in a storm-tossed sea, must learn what it means to be *me* without *you* and recognize there is no longer an *us* (at least in the physical sense). In so doing, the griever is beginning to reconstruct a world with a different, new, and hopefully fresh meaning. Will that happen overnight? It will not. The narrative of the reconstruction may go through several drafts and trial runs before a person's world is rebuilt and some sense of meaning of the loss is attained. Offering pastoral care to persons engaged in this process is not always a comfortable experience. Madeline L'Engle, as a widow, observes the following:

> *"We are not good about admitting grief, we Americans. It is embarrassing. We turn away, afraid that it might happen to us. But it is part of life, and it has to be gone through."*
>
> *Madeline L'Engle (1998, p. 299)*

Grief happens! Grief lingers! According to Ellen Goodman, *"grief is a train that doesn't run on anyone else's schedule"* (1998, p. B7). Therefore, it must be acknowledged in a healthy manner for reconstruction of life to unfold. In this chapter, we will provide some instruction concerning reconstructing life after a loss utilizing a series of five lessons developed by Robert Neimeyer of the University of Memphis contained in his book, *Lessons of Loss: A Guide to Coping* (1998).

Lesson I

> *"Grief is a personal process, one that is idiosyncratic, intimate, and inextricable from our sense of who we are."*
>
> *Robert Neimeyer (1998, p. 89)*

In essence, Neimeyer is saying that you are the only one who can be you and do your grief. It is true that others will grieve the same loss that you have experienced, but they did not have the particular relationship with the deceased that you had: similar in some ways, different in others. Furthermore, Neimeyer points out that losses *"can occasion profound shifts in our sense of who we are, as whole facets of our past that were shared with the deceased slip away from us forever, if only because no one else will ever occupy the unique position to us necessary to call them forth."* To put it simply, your life will never be the same again after the loss of a loved one, and for many, that fact is very problematic.

The death of a beloved family member, in the words of Neimeyer, *"shakes our sense of self and world"* (1998, p. 89) and causes us to respond like Sally Field in *Steel Magnolias*:

> *"Lord I wish I could understand ... I wish someone would explain this to me."*
>
> *Sally Field in Steel Magnolias*

However, when the attempts to explain fall short of one's expectations, the griever may ask: "Who am I *now*?" "What is my purpose in life?" Questions like these may surface, particularly if a mother loses her only child, and especially if she was a single parent. "Who am I without my child?" "Who am I without the future my child would provide?" However, the same can also happen in two-parent homes. During a conversation with my (SLJ) close friend, Lynn Mabe, she related that her daughter Lainie was "her life." If something were to happen to Lainie, Lynn's identity would be in serious jeopardy, even though she is the loving wife of Chris, who adores her.

In spite of the fact that any number of people grieve simultaneously for a given loss, Americans bring their common commitment to individualism to the grief process. Neimeyer states: *"No two people—not even husband and wife—can be presumed to experience the same grief in response to the same loss"* (1998, p. 91).

Grief is a personal process.

Lesson 2

> *"Grieving is something we do, not something that is done for us."*
>
> *Robert Neimeyer (1998, p. 91)*

Death can make people feel out of control, defenseless, helpless, abandoned. This is especially the case in long marriages wherein responsibilities have been clearly, perhaps traditionally, defined. Grief is that *"unwelcome intruder in our lives"* (Neimeyer, 1998, p. 91); after all, no one volunteers for grief. However, a person stands alone against it: as alone against grief as against Roger Federer (2006 champion) on Centre Court at Wimbledon. While it is true that there are many things friends and family can do for the grieving person, like in the game of singles tennis, each griever stands alone.

Because of this reality, grievers must speak up and speak out for themselves and not let others put words into their mouths. Margaret Stroebe concurs with this advice: *"... one must confront and speak of one's personal feelings and reactions to the death of the loved one"* (1992–93, p. 19). Furthermore, Neimeyer suggests that grief has to do with choices:

> *"At the most basic level we have a choice of whether to attend to the distress occasioned by our loss, to feel and explore the grief of our loved one's absence, or to dis-attend to or suppress our private pain and focus instead on adaptation to a changed external reality."*
>
> *Robert Neimeyer (1998, p. 91)*

In the midst of the sorrow and devastation people feel at the death of a loved one, there is a bewildering maze of decisions to be made. Should there be an autopsy? Which funeral home should I use? In the absence of pre-need arrangements or the deceased's wishes being clearly known, choices have to be made concerning the disposition of the body (*see* Box 11.1).

Box 11.1

View the body	or	Not view the body
Have a service	or	Not have a service
Bury	or	Cremate
Have a committal	or	Not have a committal
Earth plot	or	Mausoleum

Financial issues can and often do figure into those immediate concerns: cremation or burial; if burial, which casket? Monetary matters can continue beyond the funeral as well. "Since I can no longer afford the mortgage payments on my salary alone, what am I to do?"

Unfortunately, scenarios like this happen all too frequently. How can they be prevented? Preplanning is the key: preplanning for healthcare, retirement, college funding for children, financial resources for surviving family in case of an untimely death, an up-to-date estate plan. Pastoral care givers can and should play a significant role in helping people see the necessity of wise/careful preplanning.

There are decisions to be made in deaths resulting from "at-fault" accidents or intentional "at-fault" deaths. Many people would offer the advice of suing for damages. So, should we sue or not? Unfortunately, legal cases often continue for years before there is any resolution, satisfactory or unsatisfactory. Ironically, the "someone" who pays may be the survivor.

The choices and decisions discussed here are only a few of the many that grievers have to make. However, a goodly number of them can be helpful in the grieving process if we choose for them to be so.

Grief is something we do.

Lesson 3

"Grieving is the act of affirming or reconstructing a personal world of meaning that has been challenged by loss."

Robert Neimeyer (1998, p. 92)

This challenge has come, most definitely, without one's permission and, in some cases, without forewarning. So, the question many grievers ask is: "Where do I begin?" Frederica Mathewes-Green offers a similar set of questions for consideration:

"The only useful question in such a time is not 'why?' but 'what's next?' 'What should I do next?' 'What should be my response to this ugly event?' 'How can I bring the best out of it?'"

Frederica Mathewes-Green (1999, p. 57)

Moreover, the "ambushes" or detours that occur in the midst of that initial challenge have the potential for some continual re-challenges, thereby complicating healthy grieving by delaying the process. The following are some examples of these ambushes.

Consider the story of a recently bereaved widow who is counting on her spouse's life insurance policy proceeds to maintain the financial stability of the family. When she files the claim she learns that he borrowed heavily against the policy's cash value to pay gambling debts. In another case, the policy had lapsed for nonpayment of premiums. Would something like that issue a new challenge?

When the death is a homicide or an at-fault accident, the emotional, spiritual, and physical stakes are higher. Not only is the bereaved grieving the loss of the loved one, but also fighting with the criminal and/or civil court system. If the court case results in no conviction or if there was no arrest to begin with, the grievers remain in a "limbo" situation. It is very difficult to reconstruct a personal world of meaning in any of the situations presented.

The former scenarios are bad enough, but consider having to deal with multiple deaths as a result of violence. The Mothers' March in 2000 was an initiative of family members who experienced more than one loss due to violence. One of the mothers in that march addressed teenagers at a funeral in Kansas City with these words:

"You've got to stop the killing, so I can stop crying! Don't make another mother go through what I am going through. Stop the killing!"

How do people affirm and reconstruct meaning challenged by loss? Broadly speaking, there are two choices.

1. A griever can become the *victim* of a tragedy.
2. A griever can become the *victor* over a tragedy.

Is either of those a simple, easy task? It is most certainly not! The kind and/or number of deaths will either lessen or intensify the difficulty of assimilation or accommodation.

It is an individual choice—to grieve or not to grieve; to grieve in a healthy or unhealthy manner.

Grieving is the ongoing action of reconstructing a personal world of meaning.

Lesson 4

"We spontaneously seek opportunities to tell and retell the stories of our loss, and in so doing, recruit social validation for the changed story lines of our lives."
Robert Neimeyer (1998, p. 94)

Grief is like remodeling a house. The bereaved construct their new world by telling their stories over and over and "remodeling" them in the repeated retellings. Susan Ford Wiltshire (1994) suggests that the stories of deceased loved ones keep getting written and rewritten. For some people, the safe place to tell those stories is in grief support or aftercare groups. Other individuals see little or no value in them and reflect that sentiment in words like these: "What good does it do to keep talking about it?"

Support groups are important because they provide an opportunity for telling the story without fear of reprisal. People receive social validation from persons of a kindred spirit. These groups are a safe haven, for no one will interrupt you with, "You shouldn't feel that way." Neimeyer has something to say on the importance of expressed feelings in the grief journey:

"Feelings have a function, and are to be respected as integral to the process of meaning reconstruction, rather than controlled or eliminated as unwanted by-products of the loss itself or our 'dysfunctional' ways of thinking about it."
Robert Neimeyer (1998, p. 95)

Whether immediately or postponed, grievers reconstruct meaning through the telling and retelling of their stories.

Lesson 5

"We construct and reconstruct our identities as survivors of loss in negotiation with others."
Robert Neimeyer (1998, p. 96)

Even though grief is personal, grievers need support. Someone somewhere knows what you now need to know not just for your own survival but for the same of your family and friends. How does the bereaved find that someone? Neimeyer has this advice:

"Grievers must be active agents in negotiating the course of the post-loss adjustment."
Robert Neimeyer (1998, p. 96)

Even though it means admitting vulnerability, grievers must ask for support. Unfortunately, many of the promises of support vocalized at the visitation, funeral service, or graveside ceremony were never fulfilled. Therefore, those people with the noblest intentions to "be there" need to be reminded: "Remember what you promised to do for me at the funeral?" "I need you to help me with that now." Elizabeth Harper Neeld states that grievers need to be in communication with people whom they know care about them:

"As time goes, it will become even more important that we let our friends and family know what we need ... We should, therefore, ask ..."
Elizabeth Harper Neeld (1990, p. 48)

This is not only important for the fulfillment of the griever's present needs, but can be equally important as a way of communicating to family and/or friends what is *really* going on. Friends often talk among themselves and will ask, "How is she doing?" Then, they will share their own insights and conclude with an assessment of her condition. The friends' perceived reality of her situation may well be quite contrary to the true reality. In order to avert misperceptions, open lines of communication between the griever and the support persons are important. Such will go a long way in paving the way for that individual or individuals with whom the bereaved can feel comfortable in their grief, people with whom no pretenses exist. Neeld describes a support person as:

> *"Someone who gives total permission to grieve, who encourages us to talk as much as we wish, to cry, to show our anger; Someone who does not try to make us feel better or urge us to make the best of what has occurred or attempt to show us the good that is still present in our lives."*
>
> Elizabeth Harper Neeld (1990, p. 49)

Where does one find a person(s) like that? One's faith community is an excellent place because of the commonly shared spirituality, an important element in healthy grief. Another great source of support is someone who has experienced a similar loss. DelBene writes that the death of a close friend has given him *"a particular empathy for others whose best friends die"* (DelBene *et al.*, 1991, p. 30). How true this is.

My (SLJ) mother was a support person for and care giver with Norma Jean whose husband, Johnny, was dying with cancer. When my father became bedridden, totally unable to care for himself, Norma Jean was there day and night to care for Dad and Mom. My mother related that she did not know how she could have made it without Norma Jean. There is any number of places to recruit support. The key is in the words of Nike: *"Just do it!"*

> *"Fully engaging in mourning means that you will be a different person from the one you were before you began."*
>
> Anne Brener (1993, p. 146)

Brener's words describe the results of the willingness of a griever and support people to find common ground on which support can be given and received. Reconstruction of meaning may well be difficult, but it can happen, in large part, because we are in negotiation with others who will support, encourage, and challenge us.

To summarize this discussion, we propose the question: "What are the five lessons for reconstructing one's life after a loss?"

- **Lesson 1**: Grief is a personal process, one that is idiosyncratic, intimate, and inextricable from our sense of who we are.
- **Lesson 2**: Grieving is something we do, not something that is done for us.
- **Lesson 3**: Grieving is the act of affirming or reconstructing a personal world of meaning that has been challenged by loss.
- **Lesson 4**: Grievers spontaneously seek opportunities to tell and retell the stories of their loss, and in so doing, recruit social validation for the changed story lines of their lives.
- **Lesson 5**: Grievers construct and reconstruct their identities as survivors in negotiation with others.

We conclude this chapter by asking these questions:

- Is it possible to construct completion, gain closure?
- When is grief over?

As a griever herself, Hope Edelman outlines her discoveries about the duration of the grief process (1994):

- It is not linear.
- It is not predictable.
- It is anything but smooth and self-contained.
- It has no distinct beginning, middle or end.

As a more direct answer to the question of when is grief over, Worden offers this:

> *"When people regain an interest in life, feel more hopeful, experience gratification, and adapt to new roles."*
>
> *William Worden (1991, p. 19)*

However, he follows up that statement with these words:

> *"There is also a sense in which mourning is never finished."*
>
> *William Worden (1991, p. 19)*

In his book *The Journey Through Grief*, Wolfelt offers this sage advice about the completion of grief:

> *"Your feelings of loss will not completely disappear, yet they will soften and the intense pains of grief will become less frequent. Hope for a continued life will emerge as you are able to make commitments to the future ... The unfolding of this journey is not intended to create a return to an 'old normal' but the discovery of a 'new normal.'"*
>
> *Alan D. Wolfelt (1997a, p. 136)*

For some people, grief is a lifetime handicap. It was for Melodie Beattie:

> *"After my son died, I stayed with my grief, every gut-wrenching, heart-breaking, mind-shattering moment of it. Then I worked through my grief, finally accepting the lifetime handicap of the loss of my son."*
>
> *Melodie Beattie (1997, p. 147)*

How simple and yet profound are those words. Losing the life of someone who became a part of you is, in essence, losing a part of yourself. Therefore, you are in a certain sense challenged. As Wolfelt said, there is no return to life as it was before the loss. There has to be the discovery of life anew.

So, is there life after death? From one griever to another, yes there is. To get there, though, you must do the work of grief. You cannot go over it, under it, or around it. You must simply do it. Note these words of Dr. Valerie Yancey:

> *"Death is not a period, but a comma. Hope tells us that the present is not permanent."*
>
> *Dr. Valerie Yancey*

In her groundbreaking work of the stages of grief, Dr. Elisabeth Kubler-Ross maintained *"the one thing that usually persists through all these stages is hope"* (1969, p. 138).

A role of the pastoral care giver in ministry to the bereaved is to communicate this message of hope in a caring, supportive manner with the ultimate goal of helping to resurrect a life shattered by loss.

12

Diversity of Beliefs About End-of-Life Issues Among Differing Religions

Not all religious traditions believe the same or even similar things about dying, death, afterlife, and funeral/memorial practices. One tradition believes that death is part of the cycle of life—birth/death/rebirth—whereas another tradition believes that death is a translation from the physical life to the spiritual life. Then, one tradition believes in reincarnation, another immortality of the soul, and another resurrection of the physical body.

Furthermore, there is a divergence of beliefs on disposition of the remains of the deceased: cremation or burial, embalming or not to embalm. Moreover, funeral/memorial practices vary greatly among differing religious traditions and, sometimes, within religious traditions. There are also variations of beliefs within a specific faith tradition. In this chapter we examine widely accepted beliefs and practices surrounding end-of-life issues from the following religious traditions:

- Baha'i
- Buddhism
- Christianity
- Hinduism
- Islam
- Judaism
- Native American.

> ''People who say 'Be not afraid' are either crazy, in denial or on to something. This something is the presupposition of all religions that it is okay to die.''
>
> SLJ

Finally, in today's highly diverse societies, individuals are invited to participate in life and death moments of persons who practice a faith or spirituality different than their own traditions and experiences.

Baha'i

The Baha'i faith is a religion which had its beginnings in the mid-nineteenth century of the common era (CE) in the middle-eastern country of Iran. The founder of the Baha'i faith, Baha'u'llah, was a Persian nobleman whose name in Arabic means "The Glory of God." The sacred texts of the Baha'i faith are the writings of its founder, who in these writings emphasizes unity and oneness: God is one; all of the world's great religions are one; humanity is one.

With respect to its view of humanity, the Baha'i faith asserts that the proper understanding of human beings is spiritual in nature. The essential identity of each person is defined by an invisible, rational and everlasting soul. Furthermore, the soul grows and develops only through the individual's relationship with God, which is nurtured through prayer, knowledge of the Scriptures, moral self-discipline and service to humanity (*The Baha'is*, 1994, pp. 17, 26–27, 33). A fundamental teaching of the Baha'i faith is that believers apply divine principles to create an ever-advancing civilization based on justice, unity, and peace.

For Baha'is, the purpose of life is to know and love God, to progress spiritually, and contribute to the advancement of civilization through the practice of spiritual principles. Such is reflected in one of the three obligatory prayers for daily recitation written by Baha'u'llah:

> *"I bear witness, O my God, that thou hast created me to know Thee and to worship Thee. I testify, at this moment, to my powerlessness and to Thy might, to my poverty and to Thy wealth. There is none other God but Thee, the Help in Peril, the Self-Subsisting."*
>
> The Baha'is (1994, p. 36)

What is the Baha'i faith's perspective on dying and death? According to Baha'u'llah (in Pinchon, *Life After Death*, 1968, pp. 21 and back cover), death offers the following:

> *"The cup that is life indeed ... It conferreth the gift of everlasting life ... life hereafter is such as we are unable to describe ... I have made death a messenger of joy to thee. Wherefore dost thou grieve? I have made the light to shed on thee its splendor. Why dost thou veil thyself therefrom?"*
>
> Pinchon (1968, p. 21)

Abdu'l-Baha (in Pinchon, *Life After Death*) counsels that one should:

> *"Consider death itself the essence of life."*
>
> Pinchon (1968, p. 3)

Concerning life after death, the soul never dies. What, then, happens to the soul? Baha'u'llah explains:

> *"The world beyond is as different from this world as this world is different from that of the child while still in the womb of its mother."*
>
> The Baha'is (1994, p. 35)

This world is the place of preparation of the soul for the "world beyond" just as the womb prepares the unborn for life in the outside world. As such, heaven can be viewed, in part, as a state of intimacy with God. Conversely, hell can be perceived as a state of distance from God. The determining factor, with respect to which state one enters, is the progression or regression in one's spirituality. However, a specific understanding of the Baha'i faith's concept of the world beyond cannot be quantified. Baha'u'llah relates the following:

> *"The nature of the soul after death can never be described."*
>
> The Baha'is (1994, p. 35)

A Baha'i funeral service is open to people of all faith traditions. The primary reason for a Baha'i funeral is to honor the spiritual development and contribution of the deceased. Concerning the funeral service, the local Baha'i community's Spiritual Assembly works with the family in the planning and coordinating. The Spiritual Assembly also appoints someone, in concert with the family, to conduct the service since there is no ordained clergy in the Baha'i faith. Furthermore, the format of the service is simple; there are no rituals. In addition to music or a eulogy, if the family desires, the service consists of prayers and readings from the Baha'i sacred writings. The only required element of the service, however, is the recitation of the Prayer for the Dead (for Baha'is over the age of 15) at the gravesite by one believer, while all present stand:

> *"O my God! This is Thy servant and the son of Thy servant who hath believed in Thy signs, and set his face towards Thee, wholly detached from all except Thee. Thou art, verily, of those who show mercy the most merciful.*

> *Deal with him, O Thou Who forgivest the sins of men and concealest their faults, as beseemeth the heaven of Thy Bounty and the ocean of Thy grace. Grant him admission within the precincts of Thy transcendent mercy that was before the foundation of the earth and heaven. There is no God but Thee, the Everlasting, the Most Generous."*

> *(Let him, then, repeat six times the greeting "Allah-u-Abhah," and then repeat nineteen times each of the following verses:*

> *"We all, verily, worship God.*
> *We all, verily, bow down before God.*
> *We all, verily, are devoted unto God.*
> *We all, verily, give praise unto God.*
> *We all, verily, yield thanks unto God.*
> *We all, verily, are patient in God."*)

> *(If the dead be a woman, let him—i.e. the leader—say: "This is Thy hand-maiden and the daughter of Thy handmaiden" at the beginning of the prayer and insert the appropriate gender description thereafter.)*

Treatment of the deceased's body is more regulated, though, than the component parts of the funeral or memorial service.

- The body should be carefully washed and placed in a shroud of white cloth (silk preferably).
- Embalming is prohibited unless required by law.
- There is a prohibition against transporting the body more than one hour's journey from the place of death, even for burial.
- Cremation is prohibited.
- Burial should take place within 24 hours, if possible.
- The body can be donated for medical research as long as the laws concerning cremation and transport are strictly observed.
- Organ/tissue donation is permitted.

The grief expressed by family and friends of the deceased is related to the absence of the person's physical presence among the living. However, this separation is short-lived as the following words indicate (in *How Different Religions View Death and Afterlife*):

> *"This separation is temporal; this remoteness and sorrow is counted only by days. Thou wilt find him in the kingdom of God and thou wilt attain to the everlasting union."*

> *Johnson and McGee (1998, p. 17)*

The physical life is but the first part of an eternal existence. Furthermore, one's identity is not lost at death; souls recognize each other in the spirit world (i.e. the world beyond). Death, thus, is simply the beginning of greater things happening in the life of one's soul.

> *"The spirit of the dead will survive in the memory of the living."*
> *Quote from the epilogue of The Mission, a movie starring Robert DeNiro*

With respect to spiritual care for Baha'is in a clinical setting, ministry from clergy of other faiths is not only appropriate but welcomed. Baha'is believe that sickness can be healed through the uses of medicine and prayer. Additionally, Scripture readings from the Baha'i Sacred Writings, the Bible, the Koran, other holy books may be read to a Baha'i believer at the bedside in a hospital or some other healthcare institution. One does not need to be a clergyperson, though, to perform these ministry services (i.e. reading or praying).

Furthermore, Baha'i patients may wish to have religious objects in their hospital rooms. A picture of a nine-pointed star placed in an appropriate position is an example of one such object. Other objects could include a picture of Abdu'l-Baha, son of the Prophet Founder of the Baha'i faith, a prayer book, or other books containing Baha'i writings.

"The Prayer for the Dead" can be recited only by a Baha'i believer. However, there are other prayers which can be said by anybody on behalf of the deceased.

Two examples of these prayers were given by Abdu'l-Baha:

> *"Oh my God! O my God! Verily, thy servant, humble before the majesty of Thy divine supremacy, lowly at the door of Thy oneness, hath believed in Thee and Thy verses, hath testified to Thy word, hath been enkindled with the fire of Thy love, had been immersed in the depths of the ocean of Thy knowledge, hath been attracted by Thy breezes, hath relied upon his supplications to Thee, and hath been assured of Thy pardon and forgiveness. He had abandoned this mortal life and hath flown to the kingdom of immortality, yearning for the favor of meeting Thee.*
>
> *"Lord, glorify his station, shelter him under the pavilion of Thy supreme mercy, cause him to enter Thy glorious paradise, and perpetuate his existence in Thine exalted rose garden, that he may plunge into the sea of light in the world of mysteries.*
>
> *"Verily, Thou are the Generous, the Powerful, the Forgiver and the Bestower."*
>
> *"O my God! O Thou forgiver of sins, bestower of gifts, dispeller of afflictions!*
>
> *"Verily, I beseech Thee to forgive the sins of such as have abandoned the physical garment and have ascended to the spiritual world.*
>
> *"O my Lord! Purify them from trespasses, dispel their sorrows, and change their darkness into light. Cause them to enter the garden of happiness, cleanse them with the most pure water, and grant them to behold Thy splendors on the loftiest mount."*

Finally, these words of Abdu'l-Baha can be used as a source of encouragement for a bereaved member of the Baha'i Faith (in *How Different Religions View Death and Afterlife*):

"Whenever thou rememberest the eternal never-ending union, thou wilt be comforted and blissful."

Johnson and McGee (1998, p. 19)

Buddhism

Historians call the sixth century BCE (before the common era) the dawning of the "contemplative age." This era arose, in part, because of people's disillusionment with traditional cults and a desire to search for new forms of spirituality with emphases on individual authority, understanding, and experience. In this historical context Buddhism began.

Buddhism originated in India in the fifth century BCE in what is now known as Nepal, Siddhartha Gautama Sakyamuni's (c. 536–476 BCE) birthplace. Legend has it that as a young prince, Siddhartha faced encounters outside of his palace walls that made a lifelong impression and formed the basis for his teachings. On separate occasions, he came across a sick person, an old man, a corpse, and a holy man or wandering ascetic. He left the comfort of his family and home to seek the meaning behind these realities of sickness, aging, death, and spirituality. After a long and painful quest, he experienced his enlightenment. As a result, Siddhartha was thereafter referred to as "the Buddha," meaning "one who is awakened." During the experience of enlightenment, he formulated what was to become the core of Buddhist teachings—the Four Noble Truths:

1. All life is characterized by pain and suffering.
2. The root cause of suffering lies in the natural tendency to grasp, to cling, and to desire.
3. There is a solution to the end of suffering.
4. The method to alleviate suffering is following the Eightfold Path (Box 12.1).

Box 12.1   The Eightfold Path

1. Right understanding
2. Right thought
3. Right speech
4. Right action
5. Right effort
6. Right endeavor
7. Right mindfulness
8. Right concentration

According to Lama Chuck Stanford (1999) of the Rime Buddhist Center in Kansas City, the teachings of the Buddha were not written down until approximately 300 years after his death by the various schools of Buddhism that had evolved through the years. There are different opinions among Buddhist scholars as to the number of schools of thought within Buddhism. Some suggest two—Theravada (the oldest) and Mahayana—whereas others, along with Stanford, suggest a third major school— Vajrayana (which incorporates the teachings of the other two schools). However, the core principles of the Four Noble Truths and following the Eightfold Path are central to the beliefs and practice of Buddhists throughout the world, regardless of the schools to which they belong.

Other basic Buddhist practices include:

- meditation
- study and reflection
- practicing compassion
- cultivation of virtue which comes from following the Five Precepts:
  - avoid taking life unnecessarily
  - avoid taking others' property
  - avoid sexual misconduct
  - avoid negative speech
  - avoid intoxication.

According to Buddhist teacher Bruce Nelson (2001), Buddhism's growing appeal and rapid growth in the Western world is based on a number of factors:

- It has a rich form of spirituality.
- It emphasizes meditation and contemplative practices.
- It has an individual rather than a social/institutional focus.
- It has an ancient, magical worldview.
- Its teachings are gentle, forgiving and nondogmatic, emphasizing compassion.

Buddhism teaches that the purpose of life for any person is to end suffering in oneself and others by practicing compassion (Stanford, 1999). Thus, a genuine Buddhist would exercise loving kindness towards every human being and identify himself/herself with all, making no distinction whatsoever with regard to stature in society, color of skin, or gender. A real Buddhist is a citizen of the world who regards the whole world as the Motherland and all as brothers and sisters.

Anne C. Klein, in *How Different Religions View Death and Afterlife* (Johnson and McGee, 1998), states that dialogues of impermanence (death being the ultimate of impermanence) are at the very center of Buddhism's understanding of the human condition. These views derive from the Buddha, whose spiritual quest was initiated by his observations of suffering (Johnson and McGee, 1998, p. 47). Since a major belief of Buddhism is rebirth, a typical Buddhist works diligently to make the best use of the present life (i.e. being a morally upright, compassionate person). The reason for this mindset is that the type of one's rebirth is not guaranteed.

Fundamental to Buddhist thought about death are these concepts:

- Death is inescapable (Klein, in Johnson and McGee, 1998, p. 52).
- Death is imminent (Klein, in Johnson and McGee, 1998, p. 52).
- Death is natural (Nelson, 2001).
- Law of Karma is the concept which teaches that merit is the determining factor in one's status in rebirth (Nelson, 2001).
- Death is a temporary state between rebirths (Stanford, 1999).
- Rebirth is something to avoid (Nelson, 2001).

These last two concepts are the basis for the Buddhist philosophical preparation for death:

- Death and impermanence are part of life. If there were no death, there would be no life. Therefore, impermanence is considered to be the Source of Beauty.
- Live in the present each moment. The knowledge that change is the only constant in life can help to alleviate the desire to hold onto things.
- Clarity of mind and awareness are of utmost importance. Awareness of uncertainty when death will come can be the impetus for inspiration of spiritual effort in life.
- Escapist mentality is discouraged. It is important to see things as they really are. Therefore, there is the encouragement to meditating on life and death.
- There is a higher reality than the tangible world. Birth, life, sickness, death, rebirth are all part of the cyclical pattern of existence, part of the "Larger Harmony."

These powerful concepts can be the catalyst for intense reflection upon death and, thus, the stimulus for embarking upon spiritual practice as a means of preparing for death (Klein, in Johnson and McGee, 1998, p. 54). In that sense, Klein states:

> *"Death is religious opportunity."*
> *Anne C. Klein (in Johnson and McGee, 1998)*

In the process of dying, the senses and consciousness begin to successively wane. However, prior to this happening, family and friends are welcomed to tell their loved one good-bye and to do so without tears for the purpose of not causing guilt in the dying person. This is an extremely important consideration, for the state of mind in which one dies is a significant determining factor in the state of the subsequent rebirth (Klein, in Johnson and McGee, 1998, p. 55).

When the consciousness has gone through some deterioration and the senses begin to fade, the dying person has several visions before consciousness fully leaves the body. In humans, these stages range from 12 hours to three days (Klein, in Johnson and McGee, 1998, pp. 55–57).

- Eyesight dims causing a mirage-like vision.
- Hearing loss resulting in cessation of humming sound and internal appearance of smoke.
- Smell dysfunction signifying one is no longer cognizant of the affairs of persons with whom there was a relationship; internal vision resembles fireflies in smoke.

(All thought has now ceased. In the final four stages, there are successive visions similar to light colors suffused from dusk till dawn.)

- White moonlight.
- Red sunlight.
- Black darkness.
- White dawn—awakening into the "clear light of death."

Throughout the dying process, a religious teacher, who may be a friend or relative, often recites instructions reminding the dying person to remain calm and aware of the stage of the "clear light of death." Prayers, incense, mantra recitations, blessings of concerned individuals may also be offered for the person's benefit. The point of death, the intermediate state between death and rebirth, is a critical juncture in the life of the deceased.

For a much fuller understanding of the Buddhist concept of dying and death, Lama Stanford (1999) recommends reading *The Tibetan Book of Living and Dying* by Sogyal Rinpoche (1993). In a brief paper entitled "Guidelines for a Buddhist Funeral" (1999), Stanford discusses the precarious nature of the period between death and rebirth. Those who practice Buddhism believe that the deceased's body should not be disturbed for three days. Disturbing the body may impede the deceased's journey through the "bardo" (intermediate or temporary state). During this three-day period, it is also traditional (if practical) for individuals to meditate continually in the same room as the body. Thereafter, the body is cremated.

However, if the body is not to be disturbed for three days, this would negate any consideration of organ or tissue donation. Lama Stanford relates that he has consulted with high Lamas and Rinpoches concerning this issue. The counsel he received was favorable toward organ donation (i.e. it is good because of the expression of compassion in helping another person). Therefore, if the deceased desired to be an organ donor, the person's request should be honored.

In honoring the deceased, Buddhists typically have a funeral service (body present) and a memorial service (body not present). The funeral service is conducted as soon as possible after the death at a Buddhist center, in the home, and/or at a funeral home. At the funeral, a small shrine is built (complete with a picture of the deceased to be burned at the memorial service); flowers, candles, and incense are also present. An abbreviated service includes the following elements:

- meditation (no longer than ten minutes)
- eulogy
- explanation of Buddhist meaning of death (reference is made to various texts, for example, *The Tibetan Book of the Dead*).

The fundamental message conveyed to the bereaved is that it is important to "let go" and not cling to the deceased. The concept of "letting go" is for the purpose of aiding the deceased on his or her journey towards rebirth, whereas "hanging on" to the deceased can hinder the journey's progress. Another aid in helping the deceased on this journey is the practice of Tonglen meditation with the deceased as its object. Shortly after the semi-private funeral, the body is cremated. If there is a public memorial service, a format employed by Stanford (1999) is:

- song
- introduction (celebration of life and death)
- explanation of Buddhist concept of death
- eulogy
- meditation and reading of Sukhavati Chant (listed below)
- invitation to individuals to speak about the deceased
- poem ("I Am Not Here")
- song and concluding words.

Some of these elements would also be included in the semi-private ceremony, discussed in the previous paragraph, if there was no subsequent public service. It is also important to note that there is no prescribed order for a Buddhist funeral. The funeral services described here contain elements of Eastern and Western Buddhism utilized by Stanford.

Sukhavati Chant

> "In the profundity and brilliance of dharmakaya
> The compassion of Avalokitesvara arises.
> In the magnificent and victorious vision
> We proclaim the Jnana of Amitabha.
> You are in the state of simplicity and you are free from fetters.
> You have actually attained the fundamental enlightenment.
> Please look upon us.
> Forgive us our confusion.
> Forgive us that we have been misled by the samsaric world.
> I make offerings to you.
> I rejoice in your virtues.
> I request you to remain in our world and continue to turn the wheel of dharma.
> Namo Amitabhaya
> Samaya Tistuam
> Please accept drinking water, flowers, incense, light, perfume, food, and music.
> I praise your magnificent wisdom and power.
> You can liberate all sentient beings with one glance of your prajna and upaya.
> I request you to liberate the sentient beings who have passed and departed from
> their physical lives.
> May they be released from their samsaric fetters and attain liberation at once.
> If not so, may they attain a good human birth which is free and well favored.
> If this is not possible, may they be freed from the lower realms.
> I aspire to and worship your vision and your vow so that this Particular sentient
> being (name) and all other sentient beings may be liberated from the fetters and
> klesas, so that they may begin to overcome their mental obstacles and begin to
> understand the notion of egolessness.
> May they be free from the ayatanas.
> May they attain a state of liberation.
> May the merit of the sangha provide eternal companionship for them.
> May the blessings of the teacher lead them on their journey.
> May their relative and companions proceed with them on their journey.
> Namo Amitabhaya."

The second part of the semi-private ceremony is conducted on exactly the 49th day of the person's death, because it is the Buddhist belief that rebirth occurs 49 days after one dies. In reality, this is a ceremony of celebration. The format of the memorial service is reminiscent of the previous service 49 days earlier. One notable difference is the burning of the deceased's photograph during the recitation of the Sukhavati Chant.

We conclude this section by listing some things that Bruce Nelson (2001) provided for chaplains, other clergy, laypersons, and healthcare professionals to do and be aware of to help sick and dying Buddhist patients:

- Exhibit kindness and compassion.
- Keep the patient as pain free as possible but not to the point of diminishing clarity of thought. The proper balance is to allow for quality of life in sickness and death but also to allow for enlightenment.

- Have a natural presence; be there without an agenda.
- Be willing to listen.
- Be available.
- Be friendly and honest.
- Create a peaceful environment in order to facilitate clarity, thereby enabling the patient to work through emotional and spiritual healing.
- Allow space for the patient to work through psychological and spiritual issues.
- Be willing to share and help in any way possible, but do not be intrusive.
- Pray for the patient. All warmth and divine assistance is greatly appreciated.
- Remember the following important items concerning Buddhist patients who are dying:
  - The need is for them to let go, to become non-attached.
  - Silence and space are necessary to accomplish separation.
  - Awareness is always present, even in unconsciousness and death.
  - There may be a desire of the patient to set up a small shrine.

Finally, Buddhist understanding of life as an ongoing series of changes via birth, death, rebirth helps one not to cling to attachment of the present life. Because of this, Stanford states:

> *"May all beings be happy; may all beings be free from suffering."*
>
> Chuck Stanford (1999)

Christianity

> *"Death, where is your victory?"*
> *"Death, where is your sting?"*
> *"Death is swallowed in victory!"*
> *"I am the resurrection and the life."*
> *"He is not here; He is risen."*

These are only a small sampling of Scripture verses and songs of the Christian faith that speak of death and dying. The message which they, and the many others, convey is one of hope, assurance, comfort, and peace. Even the place where many decedents' remains are placed is not referred to in a pejorative manner (i.e. a reference to death as finality), but simply as a "place of sleep." The reference is to the word "cemetery" (derived from the Greek word *koimaomai* translated as "I sleep" or "I fall asleep"). This nomenclature for the place of burial has existed since the early centuries of the Christian era. And it should come as no surprise, for the New Testament has many references to the dead as only "being asleep."

Yet, with all of the encouraging words in the Christian Scriptures, songs, poems about death, the death of a loved one is painful, agonizing, and seemingly unbearable. For many devotees of the Christian faith, serious illness or death causes one question to be asked repeatedly.

> *"Why?"*

If God is all-good, all-loving and all-powerful, then "Why ...?" Unfortunately, in some cases there is no answer to such perplexing questions. Even so, a goodly majority of Christian believers cling to the premise and promise that a tender, gracious, caring God stands with and upholds them in difficult times, a hope reflected in the popular poem "Footprints." Truly, God is with the dying and the bereaved in the "valley of the shadow of death" offering comfort and consolation.

However, there are some within the Christian tradition who suggest that people within their same faith community are weak in the faith if they have difficulty accepting the loss of a loved one. Such is expressed in various ways:

- "He's not suffering anymore."
- "She's in a better place now."
- "Everything that happens is God's will."
- "Little Johnny will not have to endure the hardships of growing up."

In essence, people who say such things are in actuality challenging the griever, "Why are you sad?" Of course, there are many more similar clichés spoken for the purpose of "helping" the bereaved feel better, get over the loss, and get on with life. However, attempting to "cliché" grievers through emotional and spiritual suffering is to misunderstand the Christian concept of mourning the loss of a loved one. The Apostle Paul counseled that Christians do not grieve like those who have no hope. Noticeably, he is not saying they do not grieve. On the contrary, he relates that their grief is only different. As we have said previously, grief is normal and healthy. If people could understand one thing:

> *"Bereaved individuals do not want to get over the loss."*

With God's help, though, and that of other family and friends, the bereaved get through the loss. But, life will never be the same. Well then, can life ever be good again? It certainly can, although it will be different.

Now, we want to direct the discussion to various ways and means by which the dying can have a meaningful death. According to several recent studies on topics of interest to dying persons, family and faith were among the top concerns. In fact, the same concerns are true for people of virtually all races and religions.

With respect to family, several things are important. Being able to resolve unfinished relational business and address any regrets goes a long way in facilitating a peaceful death and a lack of guilt in the bereaved. Ira Byock, in *The Four Things That Matter Most: A Book About Living*, offers a five-step process of what he calls relationship completion:

1. "I forgive you."
2. "You forgive me."
3. "Thank you."
4. "I love you."
5. "Good-bye."

Think how much easier it would be to say that last "Good-bye," after giving considerable attention to the other opportunities of the process.

Another thing of importance to the dying and the bereaved is having the opportunity to celebrate the life. This time of celebration is often done around bedsides in hospitals, private residences, or nursing homes. These celebrations are often times of telling stories: upbeat, positive, and humorous. Sometimes, there is a party, even if the dying person is unable to participate. Such was the case when my (SLJ) father died. A week prior to his death, we celebrated my mother's and his beloved wife's birthday as a family around his bed. Even though Dad was semi-comatose and virtually unresponsive, he was included in the festivities.

With respect to matters of faith, many dying Christians enjoy the reading of Scripture and prayer. Here are examples of favorite texts of Scripture and a prayer on behalf of the dying person (citation is from the New Revised Standard Version of the Bible).

"The Lord is my shepherd I shall not want.
He makes me lie down in green pastures; he restores my soul.
He leads me in right paths for his name's sake.
Even though I walk through the darkest valley, I fear no evil;
for you are with me; your rod and your staff—they comfort me.
You prepare a table before me in the presence of my enemies;
you anoint my head with oil; my cup overflows.
Surely goodness and mercy shall follow me all the days of my life,
and I shall dwell in the house of the Lord my whole life long."

Psalm 23

"Do not let your hearts be troubled. Believe in God, believe also in me. In my Father's house there are many dwelling places. If it were not so, would I have told you that I go to prepare a place for you? And if I go and prepare a place for you, I will come again and will take you to myself, so that where I am, there you may be also."

John 14:1–3

"Holy and Merciful Father,
We thank you for the gift of your Son, Jesus, whom you sent to die that we might live.
We thank you also that you raised Him from the dead and that He is seated with you in heaven.
We acknowledge that you are the Lord of Death
and the Lord of Life.
We ask that you would send your holy angels to escort this your child through death into your very presence.
Give him/her peace and comfort the family who will be saddened by the loss.
In Jesus' precious name, Amen."

Additionally, it is important to some members of the Christian faith that certain sacramental rites of the church be administered (e.g. the Anointing of the Sick, Holy Communion and Baptism).

It is also customary for a prayer to be offered by a chaplain, other clergy person, or family member for those present at the time of the loved one's death. A sample prayer is as follows.

"Dear Lord,
We entrust this dear one to your care.
Receive him/her with love into your presence.
Thank you for the life he/she lived.
Comfort and strengthen this dear family in this difficult time.
In Jesus' name, Amen."

Following the death, family and friends typically gather at the home of the immediate family of the deceased. Food is often prepared and brought to the home for several days. If the funeral/memorial service is held at a church, a lunch or dinner for the family will generally be prepared and served at that location following the service and committal (if there is one). These customs do vary, though, in different communities.

A traditional way to memorialize and honor the deceased at the funeral service is by sending flowers. (Little do many people know, though, how burdensome that can be after the service for the family who then has to do something with the multitude of fresh, perishable, expensive arrangements that adorned the chapel, church, or cathedral. However, a caring funeral director, aware of this potential burden, can and will easily handle this sort of thing.) An alternative to flowers is donations to various charities or worthy causes in the name of the deceased. One thing this accomplishes is the giving of something that will live on, whereas flowers quickly wither and die.

As far as the funeral service itself, if there is one that might be deemed typical, it would be something like this:

- prayer
- congregational song(s)
- Scripture reading
- eulogy (optional)
- music solo
- sermon/homily
- prayer.

Of this prescribed order of worship, the only elements fairly well set with respect to their order in the service are the prayers and the sermon. The prayers recited will reflect a celebration of the deceased's life and a petition for comfort for the bereaved. Similarly, the sermon will also be one of celebrating the life as well as offering words of sympathy, condolence, and comfort to family and friends.

Many Christian clergy consult with the family regarding the content of the funeral service. Thus, the Scriptures usually read are those believed to be loved by the deceased. Additionally, Scriptures will be read which reflect the Christian hope of bodily resurrection and reunion with previously deceased loved ones (e.g. 1 Thessalonians 4:14–18). The songs (congregational, instrumental, and/or solo) are also selected because they are special to the deceased and family. In some Christian traditions, sacramental ordinances are integral parts of the service, such as Holy Communion and the sprinkling of Holy Water on the casket.

A graveside service, known as the committal, is also a tradition of the Christian faith community. In fact, some families choose the setting in the cemetery for the complete service, although abbreviated. Normally a committal consists of a prayer, some words of committing the deceased's body to the earth, words of consolation to the family. This service is briefer than the funeral service, generally speaking 15 minutes or less.

Concerning disposition of the deceased, either burial or cremation is permissible within the Christian faith. Certain sects within the religious tradition or individual congregational teachings, though, may have specified teachings preferring one over the other. With respect to organ and tissue donation, the decision on this issue is left to the individual's discretion.

Care for the dying and the bereaved is a communal responsibility, including both the clergy and the laity. Moreover, there is no preset time for mourning and "moving on." Once people are able to get beyond the shallowness of the clichés, healthy, lengthy grief can be embraced by the bereaved and supported by the faith community.

> *"And now abides, faith, hope, love, these three;*
> *but the greatest of these is love."*
>
> *1 Corinthians 13:13*

Hinduism

The popular conception of Hindu beliefs concerning the divine is polytheism (belief in many gods). However, according to Anand Bhattacharyya, former president of the Hindu Temple and Cultural Center of Kansas City, that understanding is not quite accurate. Hinduism can be called a monotheistic religion (belief in one god). While it is true that there are several "named" gods of the faith, they are representations or manifestations of the one Supreme Being, Brahman, which means "all-prevailing supreme consciousness." Bhattacharyya states that Brahman is the *"formless, infinite, omniscient, omnipotent, Ruler of the universe."* The gods with form are the manifestations of Brahman. To worship these manifestations is simply a more common way to know, understand, and relate to the eternal, changeless reality, called Brahman. With respect to the Hindu concept of humanity and religion, the following four things are important to remember:

1. There is unity to all of existence.
2. All religions are pathways to the same goal.
3. Mankind's real nature is divine.
4. The goal of human life is to realize this divine nature.

This divine nature is realized through the four paths of "yogas" (union with God):

1. *Karma* yoga—service to humanity.
2. *Jnana* yoga—knowledge or intuitive discernment.
3. *Raja* yoga—meditation and spiritual practice.
4. *Bhakti* yoga—love and devotion.

Therefore, one can say that it is not only what one does that is important, but also the motivation behind the action. The purpose of one's life, according to the Hindu faith, is to perform one's duties (*dharma*) to God, to society, to family, and to oneself. With respect to death, the dying person's accumulated *karma* determines what will happen after death: rebirth to a difficult life, a good life, or unity with Brahman.

Furthermore, Bhattacharyya has provided important information on the Hindu perspective on the physical body and death:

- The physical body (sometimes called gross body) is a material product, subject to origination, growth, and decay. *Atman* is the source of consciousness, the luminous Self, the divinity within the person, the "cognizer" of the psycho-physical organism. *Atman* activates the physical body through the medium of the subtle body.

- The physical body is conceived as a walled city with a number of gates within which dwells the Self, the ruler. As the ruler is distinct from the city, so is the Self distinct from the physical body.
- Just as the city collapses when its ruler departs, so the body corrupts when the Self departs from it.
- At death, the embodied Self, called *atman* (the soul), leaves only the physical body, but departs with the subtle body with all its components and the impressions of the person's *karma*.
- Death is not the end of everything.

Moreover, these concepts on *atman* are confirmed by Kathy Riegelman who compiled information on the Hindu faith for Center for Practical Bioethics' Compassion Sabbath Resource Kit. She states that the ultimate goal of life for a devotee of Hinduism is the unity of *atman* with Brahman (Cosmic Soul). For this to occur, primarily two types of disciplines—spiritual observation of moral laws and the practice of meditation—must be accomplished. Since this is often more than can be done by many people in one lifetime, these concepts are the basis for Hindu belief in reincarnation.

So, if a person is thinking of God at death, his or her *atman* will unite with Brahman and reincarnation will be averted. Thus, it is understandable why Swami Chetananda says, *"We want the person to think of God all the time."* The *Bhagavad Gita* cites these words of the Lord:

> *"What a person thinks of at death, that he attains."*
> *Nikhilananda, Bhagavad Gita (1944)*

In order for the dying person's *atman* to unite with Brahman, though, the support and spiritual encouragement of family and friends is of great help. It is extremely helpful for spiritual care givers to call the patient's attention to God using a variety of methods:

- Placing pictures of the individual's spiritual Guru (i.e. spiritual teacher), whether alive or dead, in front of the bed.
- Utilizing audio/videotapes of holy subject matter, such as lectures on spiritual life.
- Playing devotional songs, called *bhajans.* (The songs should be in Hindi or the mother tongue of the patient.)
- Reading selected portions of holy books (e.g. the *Bhagavad Gita*, *Ramayana*, or the *Gospel of Sri Ramakrishna*, all of which can be in English, Hindi, or the patient's mother tongue).
- Encouraging the dying person to recite his or her mantrum repeatedly.
- Placing Ganges (holy) water into the patient's mouth. (Household tap water, when purified with mantrum, is acceptable for use because it would be difficult to obtain water from India's Ganges River.)

The sole purpose for these and other activities, according to Riegelman, is to help the person die "heroically," not in fear. Constant reminders to the dying person that *atman* is a part of God who never dies can greatly enhance the person's ability to die in peace and tranquility. Furthermore, the family of the dying person can call the priest of the local Hindu Temple to perform some of these activities. The priest will come to the bedside of the dying person anytime outside the Temple's open hours. In addition, he will chant *Shanti* Mantra (peace chant) or chant from other Scriptures. Moreover, if at all possible, the dying person should be moved to a private room to allow spiritual care givers to conduct spiritual practices at the time of death. These care givers can include family members, friends, priests of local Hindu temples, swamis (religious leaders) of local Vedanta Societies (philosophical Hindu sect), nurses, chaplains, or other healthcare professionals.

There are also other things that family/friends (Hindu or non-Hindu) and even healthcare and pastoral care providers can do to help the person have a peaceful death. For example, flowers can be brought in to add fragrance and color to the room. Another important thing to do is to fulfill the wishes of the dying for *prasad* (food dedicated to the Lord), for example, fruits or any food that a patient can eat or wants to eat. One source of *prasad* would be the local Hindu Temple. Those interested in helping the patient achieve a meaningful death should also attempt to cheer the dying (humor is helpful and advisable) and gently touch the head and arms of the individual as gestures of love and affection.

According to Bhattacharyya, non-Hindus can and are welcome to render many of these caring acts to a Hindu at the end of life. If nothing else, a non-Hindu interested in providing care for a dying person can, at the very least, facilitate many of these end-of-life merciful acts. However, for any care giver (Hindu or non-Hindu) to be effective, he or she must be spiritually inclined.

At the point of death, the Hindu faith teaches that if the dying person prays with utmost sincerity, his or her spiritual Guru will appear in visionary form. The importance of this experience (and the preceding ministry, which greatly enhances the likelihood of the spiritual encounter) cannot be overstated. Hinduism teaches that the epiphany of the Spiritual Guru will eradicate all of the patient's worldly desires. Therefore, there is no need for reincarnation. The ultimate goal of life has been attained: Eternal union with Brahman.

After a person dies, it is customary for a priest to come to the funeral home and perform various final rituals called *Antima Kriya:*

- Spread flowers on the deceased's body in the casket.
- Chant mantras from Scripture.
- Sprinkle holy water on the deceased.

It is preferred, but not mandatory, that a priest officiate or even participate in the funeral service. Other participants are strictly at the discretion of the family. Thus, there are several options for consideration with respect to funeral services:

- Priest alone performing prescribed rituals.
- Priest in concert with family/friends performing the service.
- Family and friends performing the service, which may include singing devotional songs, reading from Scripture, or eulogizing the deceased.

With respect to the length of the various services, if a priest is involved in the funeral proceedings, one can expect the entire service to last approximately two hours. On the other hand, if only family and friends conduct the funeral, the length of the service is approximately one hour.

Typically, the funeral service will be held one to three days following the death. After the funeral, the body is cremated and the cremated remains are placed in an urn for keeping, mixing with river water, or scattering, if the family desires. According to Bhattacharyya, many people of the Hindu faith will select a funeral home with a crematory on the premises. A family may decide to cremate the body coupled with a short funeral service, with or without the priest's presence. A few days thereafter, a memorial service would be conducted. Family and friends, who may do any or all of the following things, would perform this memorial service:

- sing devotional songs
- read selected texts from the Scripture
- share stories about the deceased.

He states that decisions regarding organ and tissue donation are personal. If a person decides to provide gifts of life and life enhancement to other people at the time of his or her death, it would not be contrary to basic teachings of Hindu faith. In fact, it would be a good deed. Bhattacharyya concludes:

"Organ and/or tissue donation would be positive karma."

The responsibility rests with friends and family for the care for the grieving and the bereaved (before and after the funeral), not with the priest. Even though it is known that *atman* is eternal (i.e. the soul never dies), loved ones of the deceased experience grief over the loss of his or her physical presence among them. Hinduism, thus, considers grief to be healthy for one's emotional health and encourages people to express their grief. To facilitate the initiation of the grief process and wishing well for the departed soul, for several days after the funeral, people are invited to the home of the deceased for the singing of devotional songs and to offer multiple other acts of kindness for the bereaved.

The following principles are important for care givers to keep in mind with respect to providing grief support and how Hindus typically mourn the loss of a loved one.

- At the time of death always expect the nearest family members, especially women, to weep loudly as an expression of grief.
- The body should be cremated within 24 hours. However, this is always not possible due to:
  - scheduling a funeral service may take time
  - the priest may not be available at short notice
  - some waiting time may be required for close relatives to arrive before the funeral service
  - if organ donation is permitted, allow additional time.
- Appropriate ways to support the bereaved:
  - Visit the grief-stricken family and offer any kind of help to the family, such as bringing cooked food, buying urgent needs, etc.
  - Hug the bereaved family members. Note: Hindu tradition generally does not allow hugging between opposite genders.
  - Offer eulogy during the funeral service, if you knew the deceased person well.
  - At the end of the service, the priest or the family may ask guests to offer their last respects to the deceased. This may involve placing a flower near the feet of the body laid in an open casket for viewing. The body is cremated as soon as possible after the funeral service.
- Post funeral service (*Shraddha*):
  - The relatives of the dead person are 'impure' (*Asauch*) for ten days.

- During this time the bereaved family sings devotional songs with friends and relatives, does not receive or give any gifts, and eats simple food. Male members do not shave, or cut hair.
- After ten days (12 days in some traditions) a ceremony called *shraddha* is performed by the family (generally by the son) with the help of a priest to help the departed soul rest in peace.
- Anniversary ritual (*Tarpan*): Each year in autumn, the living sons in many Hindu families give oblation of water to the ancestors of three generations as an act of remembrance performed to satisfy the departed ancestors.

Before concluding, we want to offer some words of counsel for healthcare providers in institutional settings regarding the spiritual care of a critically ill or dying Hindu patient. According to Bhattacharyya, it would be most helpful for the staff to provide an atmosphere conducive for the performance of various rituals, which are of utmost importance for the individual's spiritual and emotional well-being at this most critical juncture in the cycle of life.

Finally, throughout this discussion, we have made mention of mantras, prayers, Scriptures, and songs. In order to enable non-Hindus to have a ministry of caring with a dying Hindu person, we have provided a sample listing of the various readings, which can be utilized unto that end.

Mantra

> ''Shri Ram Jai Ram Jai Jai Ram
> Shri Ram Jai Ram Jai Jai Ram
> Raghupati Raghav Raja Ram
> Patit Pavan Sita Ram
> Om namah Shivaya Om nama Shivayah
> Om namah Shivaya Om nama Shivayah''

Prayer for Direction and Blessing of a Dying Person

> ''The door of the True is covered with a golden disk. Open it O Pushan, that we may see the nature of the true. O Pushan, only seer, O Yama, (judge), O Surya (sun), son of Projapati, spread your rays and gather them! I see the light, which is your fairest for I myself am He!
>
> My breath to the air, to the immortal! My body ends in ashes.
> Om! Mind remember! Remember your deeds!
>
> Agni, lead us on to prosperity by a good path. O God, you know all things! Keep crooked evil far from us, and we shall offer you the fullest praise!''

Scripture Verses from Chapter Two of the Bhavagad Gita Emphasizing Immortality of the Soul

> ''Never was there a time when I did not exist, nor you, nor these kings of men. Never will there be a time hereafter when any of us shall cease to be.'' (II, 12)

"It (the Soul) is never born, nor does It ever die, nor, having once been, does It again cease to be. Unborn, eternal, permanent, and primeval, It is not slain when the body is slain." (II, 20)

"The Self, which dwells in all bodies, can never be slain. Wherefore you should not mourn for any creature." (II, 30)

Devotional Song

"When we have fallen in love with Ram, why should we cultivate attachment with the world? When we have found the shelter of the Lord, why to efface ourselves? When Lord Ram is residing in the temple of our heart, what is the use of taking bath in sacred places outside? When He is permeating everything, what is the use of going to the temple door? When there is absolutely nothing without Ram, what is the use of forgetting oneself in the illusions of the heart? When the stream of love has started flowing, what is the use of going in search of Ram? When the perfect teacher has been found, where else to find an abode? When O mind! You remember the Lord constantly; it is the same thing as being absorbed in Ram. When we have fallen in love with Ram, why to remain attached to the world?"

"Lead me from untruth to truth, lead me from darkness unto light, lead me from death unto immortality."

Such is the desire of every devotee of the Hindu faith.

Islam

According to Imam (the Islamic title for clergy) Yusaf H. Hasan, the word "Islam" (derived from the Arabic root *SLM*) means peace, purity, obedience, and submission. Based on the last two of these four descriptive nouns, a devotee of Islamic faith submits his or her will in obedience to God. Muslims believe that Islam started with the first man, Adam, and the first woman, Eve. However, as a religious tradition, Islam had its official beginning in 622 CE by means of the adoption of divine revelation from God through the Prophet Muhammad (the last prophet in the lineage of the prophets of God), who preached the words he received until his death in 632. The revealed message was then recorded by Muslim believers and collected into a document entitled the *Qur'an* (also spelled Koran), the Holy Book of Islam.

The main tenets, with respect to duties and responsibilities of adherents of Islam, are generally understood to be five in number (Jane Idleman Smith cited in Johnson and McGee, 1998, pp. 134–135):

1. Verbalizing the *Shahadah*, the basic testimony of faith, which is "there is no God but God and Muhammad is the Prophet of God."
2. Participating in the *Salat* (public prayer) at five regularly scheduled times during the day.
3. Participating in the *Saum* (fast) observed for consecutive days during the annual month of Ramadan, a total fast from dawn to dusk for able-bodied adults.
4. Sharing of one's material goods with the community's needy through the *Zakat* (the paying of the alms-tax).

5. Making the *Hajj*, the great pilgrimage to Mecca and Medina at least once during one's lifetime.

With respect to illness, dying, and death, these common occurrences in life are as natural and normal as birth. Muslims acknowledge this and affirm that illness and death are inevitable parts of life (Hasan). Similarly, A. Rauf Mir, MD, (2001) states that death is a fact of life of which everyone should be aware because every person will encounter the loss of a friend or loved one. Death is a natural transition in life from which no one escapes. This is confirmed by the words of Allah stated in the *Qur'an*:

> *"Verily, every soul shall taste death; and only on the Day of Judgment shall you be paid your full recompense."*

> *Qur'an (3:185)*

Concerning sickness, Muslims believe that suffering from an illness causes God to discard or forgive the sins of the one stricken with infirmity. The journey through this earthly life contains illness and other hardships which remove some of people's sins (Hasan). However, sickness is not a curse and seeking the best medical treatment available is a mandatory obligation. Moreover, Islam teaches that the worldly existence is the soil in which individuals can sow, cultivate, and grow the good fruits of the afterlife. From the Islamic perspective, then, illness is not viewed in a negative light. Death, theologically at least, is also viewed positively because of the blessed hope of the resurrection of the body to a time of happiness and bliss in heaven for the faithful. Because of the truth of this latter statement, Dr. Mir (2001) relates that there are certain recommended procedures that one in the presence of the dying can do to help make the positive transition to the Afterlife:

- Kindly remind the dying person to remember and think well of Allah, his Creator, and believe that the Afterlife is real and true.
- Help the dying person not to despair of Allah's mercy but to ask Allah for his forgiveness. (This statement is validated by the following citations from Aisha—the wife of the Prophet Muhammad, "may the peace and blessings of Allah be upon him and may God be pleased with her"—and Imams Muslim and Bukhari.)

> *"Aisha reported the Prophet as saying: 'Whoever likes to meet Allah, Allah likes to meet him. But whoever dislikes to meet Allah, Allah dislikes to meet Him.'"*

> *"Aisha said, 'O Prophet of Allah, is it the hate of death?' He said, 'But when the believer is given the good news of the Mercy of Allah, His blessing and His heaven, he likes to meet Allah and Allah likes to meet him. When the unbeliever is given the news of torture and curse of Allah, he dislikes meeting Allah and Allah dislikes meeting him.'"*

- Help the dying not to wish to hasten the death because of the pain and suffering being endured. On the contrary, the person should ask Allah to give life if it would be good or to end life if that would be better.
- Help the dying person by reminding him to pay his debts. If he is currently not able to do so, he can make request of those present to do so or write in his will that all debts are to be paid from his wealth.

- Help the dying person by reminding him to write his will if he has not already done so.
- Help the dying by reminding him to say the *Shahadah*, the basic testimony of faith.

Mir (2001) continues by stating that there are other things those present can do on behalf of the dying person:

- Do not say anything except prayers and good things.
- Pray for the dying person and ask Allah to make his passing easy and to forgive his sins.
- Position the dying person such that the *Qibla* (direction of Makkah, i.e. Mecca) is on his right side.
- Recite verses from the *Qur'an*, especially *Surah Yasin* (Chapter 36).

However, when one witnesses or learns of someone's death, the words of the *Qur'an* 2:156–157 should be recited:

> *''Verily we belong to Allah and truly to Him shall we return.''*
> *Qur'an (2:156–157)*

Furthermore, the following are recommended procedures for people present with the deceased:

- Close the eyes of the deceased.
- Cover the person completely.
- Pray for forgiveness for the deceased person.
- Settle the deceased's debts, if any. (This is the role of family and/or friends.)
- Prepare the body for burial without unnecessary delay. (This function can only be done by a Muslim.)

Moreover, there are five primary elements to the preparation of a Muslim's body for disposition to be completed only by Muslims.

1. *Ghusl* (washing of the body).
2. *Kafan* (wrapping the body with a plain linen or cotton cloth).
3. *Salah al-Janaza* (formal funeral prayers).
4. *Janazah* (funeral procession).
5. Burial in a properly prepared grave.

The washing of the body is very important because cleanliness and ritual purification are fundamental principles in Islam. The washing can be performed at the place of death, at the deceased's home or in a special place outside of a mosque. Prayer and recitation of verses from the *Qur'an* are an integral part of the washing ceremony. Embalming, though, is not practiced because it is believed that the body, which is perishable, should not be impeded from returning to the earth. Following the ritual washing, the body is dried, carefully wrapped in a plain white cloth, and placed in a simple casket for transport to the place of burial (Johnson and McGee, 1998, p. 136).

Mir (2001) has provided an example of a funeral prayer:

> *''O Allah! [deceased's name] is in Your presence. Please save [him/her] the disturbance and torture of the grave. You are the one who forgives. O Allah! Forgive [his/her] sins and bestow Your mercy on [him/her]. You are Most*

Merciful, Most Forgiving. O Allah! Forgive those who are living and those who have died, our young and old, male and female, present and absent. O Allah! Those of us whom You have kept alive, keep us on the path of Islam, and those who die, let them die with faith ...''

The funeral procession is the final journey which completes *this* life. In order to speed decomposition, the body is usually removed from the casket and placed in a prepared burial site facing the East, towards Mecca (Hasan). Another reason for not having elaborate caskets and/or vaults is the expense. The money that is saved can be used to pay the deceased's debts or for contributions to things of a charitable nature (Mir). After the body is lowered, members of the Muslim community shovel dirt into the grave. Following the committal service, candy is distributed to sym-bolize the removal of the ''bitter taste of death'' from one's mouth (Hasan). According to Mir (2001), the candy distribution has no basis in the Islamic faith, but is simply a cultural custom in some communities.

How important is it that the five procedures enumerated and explained above be accomplished? Mir counsels that:

''Washing and burying the deceased is obligatory upon Muslims ... if some members (of the Muslim community) take the responsibility of doing it, the need is fulfilled. If no one fulfills it, then all Muslims will be held accountable before Allah.''

Mir (2001)

One additional important item to mention about the disposition of the body regards cremation. Because of the belief that the body is to be handled with extreme care and the understanding that fire is used by God for judgment upon the sinful, cremation is forbidden (Johnson and McGee, 1998, p. 136). Since cremation is viewed with such disdain, *it would be offensive to a Muslim to even ask about the option of cremation* (Mir, 2001). With respect to organ and tissue donation, Islamic scholars have ruled in favor of such due to the overall good it achieves. Consider the following words contained in the *Qur'an*:

''And if anyone saved a life, it would be as if he saved the whole people.''

Qur'an (5:35)

However, tissue, bones, eyes, major organs, or any viable body component pro-cured for transplantation must be used immediately and not placed in storage. The choice, though, to donate or not is an individual one, as in many other faith traditions.

Preparing food for the bereaved family is strongly encouraged, for it is a difficult time for those who lose a loved one. Communal support is, therefore, appreciated and helpful. Weeping is permissible in expressing sorrow over the loss. However, wailing and overtly loud crying are not sanctioned. With respect to the period of formal mourning, it is not to exceed three days (Mir, 2001). The community of faith is to take comfort in the fact that the deceased is in the care of Allah (Johnson and McGee, 1998, p. 137). Concerning the marking of the grave for identification purposes, a simple marker may be placed thereon, but the marker is not to be raised above one foot.

What additional things can chaplains, healthcare workers, or other non-Muslim individuals do for dying patients and bereaved families in institutional settings? Mir

(2001) says, *"Be available to offer assistance—make phone calls to the appropriate people, be sensitive to the situation."* He also suggests that it would be helpful if a private room could be made available for times of prayer by Muslims, who kneel on rugs.

There are several other things of which healthcare professionals should be aware when caring for Muslim patients (Mir, 2001):

- Blood transfusions are acceptable to those of the Islamic faith.
- Euthanasia in any form is against the teachings of Islam: Suicide, including even physician-assisted suicide.
- Withholding or withdrawing life-sustaining therapy is acceptable and appropriate treatment.
- There is nothing in the teachings of the faith to suggest the use of "heroic measures" to prolong death.
- Autopsies are to be performed for only three reasons:
  1. forensic necessity
  2. disease identification
  3. learning opportunity.
- Care at home for the dying is preferable to Muslims.
- Healthcare professionals of the same sex as the patient are preferred.
- Modesty is very important to Muslims. When a code or any procedure is being performed, care should be given to covering the "private parts" as much as possible.

Mir (2001) offers one final reminder of an Islamic fundamental teaching. The worldly life is the soil in which an individual can cultivate the fruits of the afterlife. The Prophet ("may the peace and blessing of Allah be upon him") taught the following as reported by Imam Muslim:

> *"When the son of Adam dies, his/her deeds will be discontinued except for three: a charity that continues giving (i.e. a school, a hospital), some knowledge that continues to benefit (e.g. by being passed from one person to another), or a pious child that prays for him/her."*

Judaism

Judaism is not unlike other religious traditions with respect to diversity of beliefs and practices of its various sects. Rabbi Joshua D. Kreindler (2000), former chaplain of the Jewish Federation of Broward County, Florida, confirms the diversity among those who practice Judaism:

> *"Certain beliefs and practices may be different among Orthodox, Conservative and Reform Jews."*
>
> *Rabbi Joshua D. Kreindler (2000)*

Because it is beyond the scope of this work to present all of the differing perspectives of beliefs and practices within Judaism, our intention is to present the more commonly held, traditional beliefs of the Jewish faith. Nina Shik (RN, MSN, CIC, Clinical Nurse Specialist), formerly of Shawnee Mission Medical Center, was of great help in providing us with considerable information, as well as information from Rabbi A. R. Scheinerman and Tracey R. Rich. Of significant help as well was

Rabbi Kreindler. In an unpublished paper, "Jewish Tradition and Laws Concerning Death and Mourning" (2000), he delineates quite clearly and succinctly the basic elements of Jewish belief and practice regarding life, death, afterlife, funeral practices, periods of mourning, hope, and communal opportunities for remembrance of the deceased.

End-of-life issues (death, funeral practices, grief, etc.) Kreindler (2000) contends, must be understood in the Jewish concept of life. Furthermore, the overall content of this section adheres closely, with minor deviations, to the outline of his paper.

The purpose of Israel's existence is to show and prove the holiness of God. In order to fulfill her purpose as a "Holy Nation" (the basis of the covenant between Abraham and God), Israel was to remain loyal to the teachings of Torah. According to Holy Scripture, humans were made in the image of the one invisible, powerful and mysterious God, and the world was created for people to serve God (Genesis 1:26; 2:7, 15; Isaiah 45:23). Therefore, life is highly valued among people of the Jewish faith, and such is reflected in the Talmud: *"Whoever saves one life, it is as if he has saved an entire world"* (Tractate Sanhedrin. Folo 45 a). Furthermore, Rich (1996) says that of the 613 commandments, *only* the prohibitions against murder, idolatry, incest, and adultery are so important that they cannot be violated to save a life. Saving one's own life, or that of another, takes precedence even above the observance of the Sabbath.

Generally speaking, discussions about organ/tissue donation require rabbinical consultations. When organ and/or tissue donation can save a life or improve one's health, it is permitted. Judaism expressly teaches that saving a human life takes precedence over maintaining the sanctity of the human body. Therefore, to donate any organs and/or tissue is considered to be a *mitzvah* (good deed).

> *"Death is as natural as life. It's part of the deal we made."*
> *Morrie Schwartz in Tuesdays with Morrie (Albom, 1997, p. 172)*

Because of this intense valuation of life, one would expect that illness and death would be feared and considered tragic when they occur. However, in Judaism, illness and death are considered to be natural parts of the life cycle. They, like life, are part of God's plan. Even though it is not known why God allows people to suffer, Jewish belief is that ultimately it does have meaning. This concept of death is consistent with the first of Kreindler's (2000) two reasons for death entering the world:

1. God's desire for humanity to return to the earth from which it was formed; and
2. the result of the first humans' sin of eating of the forbidden fruit.

Concerning his latter reason, the belief of the Creator as merciful and forgiving in conjunction with the belief of an afterlife dispel the attitude of distaste for death.

> *"To everything there is a season, and a time to every purpose under heaven—A time to be born, a time to die ..."*
>
> *Ecclesiastes 3:1–2*

With respect to the afterlife, traditional Judaism believes that death is not the end of human existence. However, because the adherents of the Jewish faith are primarily focused on life in the present and how to live it, the texts discussing the afterlife are not plentiful. Nevertheless, there are teachings that are unambiguous. *"Many of them that sleep in the dust of the earth shall awake, some to everlasting life, and some to reproaches and everlasting abhorrence"* (Daniel 12:2). Similarly, the great Jewish philosopher Maimonides writes this as Principle 13 of his Thirteen Principles of the Faith: *"I believe with perfect faith that the Resurrection will take place when God wills it."*

Belief in resurrection of the body, though, is not universal in Judaism. Some Jews reject this notion, opting for belief in a spiritual, not physical, afterlife. Alternatively, belief in reincarnation is a commonly held belief among mystically inclined Jewish sects. For many Jews, the concept of an afterlife is not a motivation in life. The goal is to make *this* life better, not to attain a better life in the "hereafter." However, certain things in Jewish life are eternal: one's soul, memories and acts of righteousness. Even though there is little unanimity among the differing Jewish traditions about the afterlife, there seems to be a consensus on one thing: the prospect of the messianic age, a time referred to in Hebrew texts as *olam ha-ba*—the world to come—a term used to reference the physical and/or spiritual afterlife (Rich, 1996).

Rabbi Scheinerman (2000) points to two overriding principles that govern the Jewish approach to death and mourning:

1. *kavod ha-met* or honoring the dead (i.e. treating the body with respect and care from the time of death until the burial is completed); and
2. the view that death is a natural process (a concept previously mentioned).

Concerning the former principle, it is customary to wash the body in preparation for burial. This process is called *taharah* (purification). After the ritual of purification, the body is dressed in a simple, plain linen shroud called *tachrichim*. Some people, though, may prefer that the deceased be wrapped in his or her *tallit* (prayer shawl), minus the *tzitzit* (corner fringes), which symbolizes that the *tallit* can no longer be used for prayer. However, since Jewish tradition encourages simplicity in burial (all equal before God), a plain wooden coffin with the deceased wrapped in the plain linen shroud is considered quite appropriate.

We might interject at this point several other important considerations regarding treatment of and disposition of the body (Rich, 1996):

- The body must not be cremated because it prevents the return of the body to its natural state (considered an individual choice for Reform Jews).
- The body is not to be embalmed because it is considered as mutilation to the body (individual choice for Reform Jews).
- Autopsies are discouraged as desecration of the body; they are permitted, though, if a life may be saved or required by law.
- The body is never displayed at funerals because exposing a dead body is considered disrespectful (i.e. looking down upon a person who is defenseless). Moreover, many Jews will not view the corpse if they attend the visitation of a non-Jew.
- The deceased is buried in a wooden coffin which hastens decomposition of the body back to the earth.

As a sign of respect, the body is not left alone until after the burial. *Shomerim* are individuals charged with the responsibility of watching over the body. During this time, often a candle is lit at the head of the body and the *shomer* (guard or keeper) recites psalms.

> *"We are not alone when we are born, and should not be alone when we die."*
> *Nina Shik*

Furthermore, when an *avel* (mourner) has lost a parent, sibling, spouse, or child, it is traditional that the initial grief be expressed by tearing one's clothing, although modified by some to the tearing of ribbons pinned to one's clothing. This is accompanied by reciting the following blessing: *"Blessed are You, Lord our God, Ruler of the Universe, the True Judge."* According to Kreindler (2000), this ritual helps the family focus on the death and begins the process of accepting God's taking the life of a close relative. From the time of death until after the funeral, the family does not receive visitors. Their focus is upon caring for the body and planning the funeral. Moreover, the rabbi is often among the first to hear of the death; he or she then goes to the home of the mourners to assess their well-being, perhaps participate in the *keriyah* ritual, and assist in funeral planning. Generally speaking, the funeral service is conducted within 24 hours of the death, because the Scriptures state: *"Bury him the same day ... his body shall not remain all night."* There are special circumstances (e.g. on Sabbath and on Jewish Holidays, requirement for an autopsy, relatives traveling from out of town, etc.) that would allow for a delay of up to three days.

Scheinerman (2000) relates that the funeral service may take place in a funeral home chapel, in the synagogue or at the cemetery (flowers and music discouraged). In many communities a simple graveside service is the norm. Kreindler (2000) states that after the immediate family and friends congregate at the cemetery, the coffin is slowly and solemnly brought to the gravesite. At this juncture, Psalm 91 is recited which helps those gathered see the need for reflection, repentance, and contemplation of their own mortality.

Prior to the actual burial, the rabbi, family and friends offer eulogies for two reasons (Kreindler, 2000):

1. Jewish tradition maintains that the deceased is judged before and after burial—thus, the more positive things spoken at that time, all the better for the state of the soul; and
2. the eulogy highlights the family's and community's loss, thereby accelerating active grieving essential to the healing process.

Following the eulogies as the mourners stand or sit around the gravesite, the coffin is lowered into the grave while the prayer, *"God, Abundant in Mercy,"* is chanted. When the coffin touches the bottom of the grave, it is traditional for mourners to shovel dirt into the grave as a *mitzvah* (good deed) and last commandment performed on behalf of the deceased (Kreindler, 2000). The back of a shovel is used to suggest that this act of using a shovel is different from other occasions for its use. Further-more, this practice is related to the primitive concept of "guarding" against the return of ghosts to the deceased. The shovel is not passed from person to person. After one person uses the shovel, it is placed in the dirt where it is retrieved by another and so forth. Kreindler (2000) relates that this ritual act dismisses any possibility of denial on the part of the family. The loved one is dead (Scheinerman, 2000).

At this point in the service, the Mourner's Kaddish (from the Hebrew word for holy) is recited. Amazingly, this prayer contains nothing related to death or mourning. On the contrary, it is a prayer of praise to God. Why, then, would people recite Kaddish at a time when it would be normal to expect grievers' faith to waiver or to express anger at God? Because of the probability of such happening, Judaism requires mourners to recite Kaddish publicly for two reasons:

1. to reaffirm one's faith in God despite the loss; and
2. to insure the merit of the deceased in the eyes of God.

At the conclusion of the graveside ritual, both Kreindler (2000) and Scheinerman (2000) state that two parallel lines of those present are formed through which the mourners walk to the sound of *"May you be comforted among the mourners of Zion and Jerusalem."* Prior to leaving the cemetery, some will engage in the ritual hand washing as a symbol of purification, after which the following verse is recited: *"May death be swallowed up forever, and may the Lord God wipe away the tears from every face and remove the mocking of God's people from throughout the world, for the Lord has spoken."* Then, depending on the locale, the mourners sit in the cemetery chapel as a prelude to the start of the formal grieving process (Kreindler, 2000). Still others will participate in the purification ritual of hand washing before entering the family home upon returning from the cemetery (Scheinerman, 2000). This ritual is an act of purification from association with a dead body and also, according to ancient belief, to purify the living from unclean demons.

The Jewish customs and laws following the funeral have two purposes:

1. to honor the deceased
2. to help the living.

Concerning those two purposes, Jewish mourning practices can be broken up into three periods of decreasing intensity (Rich, 1996), which structure the mourners' lives by helping them to gradually, yet steadily, and gently return to normal activities of life (Scheinerman, 2000):

1. *Shiva* begins on the day of the burial and continues until the morning of the seventh day after burial.
2. *Sheloshim* follows *Shiva* and continues through the thirtieth day counting from the burial.
3. *Avelut* follows *sheloshim* and continues for 11 months.

Shiva

This seven-day period begins with a *seudat havra'ah*, a meal of consolation, provided by relatives, friends, and neighbors immediately following the funeral (Scheinerman, 2000). The meal consists of eggs, which symbolize the elliptical nature of life (life then death), and lentils, which symbolize the mourners' inability to speak because the lentil has no opening in its shell (Kreindler, 2000). Traditionally, the mourners will sit through this period for seven days (rising only for the Sabbath and any other festivals which may intervene), and some will even sit on low stools, symbolizing their suffering at the present time. During this time, the grievers are to abstain from all work and remain home to receive visitors who view their services of consolation as meritorious. Furthermore, since mourners are not permitted to do any work (e.g. cooking), visitors bring food, not only to feed the grievers but guests as well. On a daily basis, *minyanim* (quorums of at least ten men in Orthodox circles) are organized to say morning, afternoon, and evening prayers in the mourners' home. During the interim between prayers, Bible or Talmud is studied, Psalms are recited, and people visit. Of course, Kaddish is recited daily also. The mourners honor the deceased by reminiscing, remembering, and recapturing memories of their deceased loved one. On the final day of *shiva* and after the morning prayers, the grievers are told, *"May you be comforted among the mourners of Zion and Jerusalem."*

After this, they may leave the house. However, they may not return to work or school until the next day (Kreindler, 2000).

Sheloshim

During this 30-day period (of which *shiva* is a part) following the burial, grievers do not get haircuts, buy new clothes, attend the festive part of circumcisions, weddings or Bar Mitzvahs (Kreindler, 2000), go to movies, parties, listen to music, or watch television (Rich, 1996; Scheinerman, 2000). Some, though, will listen to news on the radio (Kreindler, 2000). However, the mourners may return to work and school, and they continue to recite Kaddish daily.

Avelut

This period of mourning begins 30 days after the death and continues for 11 additional months. During this time, the grievers avoid parties, celebrations, theater, and concerts (Rich, 1996). Kaddish, however, is recited daily for only the first ten months of this period (for a total of 11 months following the burial). Why is this the case? According to Jewish tradition, the deceased's soul must spend some time purifying itself before it can enter *olam ha-ba* (the world to come) and the maximum time of purification for the most evil of people is 12 months. Therefore, to recite Kaddish for the full 12-month period of mourning would imply that the deceased was a very evil person. To avoid such an implication, then, the rabbis decreed that Kaddish should be recited for only 11 months (Rich, 1996).

Following *avelut*, the period of formal mourning concludes with the unveiling of the grave marker, accompanied by the chanting of memorial prayers and reciting Kaddish. Furthermore, the mourners, who are accompanied by the rabbi, or family and friends, take a walk to symbolize that life continues even after death (Kreindler, 2000). Now, while it is more common to unveil the grave marker at the culmination of *avelut*, some communities have the unveiling prior to the conclusion of the year of mourning; other communities do not have the unveiling until after the year has past. Local custom is the determining factor (Scheinerman, 2000).

Formal communal acknowledgments of the deceased, though, do not end with the ceremony of unveiling the grave marker. There are others:

- the annual anniversary of the loved one's death called *yahrzeit*
- at Yom Kippur and several festivals during a memorial service known as *yizkor.*

On *yahrzeit*, it is customary to light a candle in memory of the deceased and attend a synagogue service to recite Kaddish (Scheinerman, 2000). Furthermore, if the mourners are European or American Jews, they might fast and give charity in memory of their deceased loved ones and visit the cemetery. If the mourners are of the Chassidic sect, a feast is held as a way to express joy that the deceased's soul has ascended to a higher level in Paradise. In addition, Sephardic Jews (from Africa and Asia) have a feast for celebration of the same (Kreindler, 2000).

Yizkor, the memorial service on Yom Kippur (the highest holy day in Judaism) and during festivals like Passover and Tabernacles, is a time when the memory of deceased loved ones is evoked, along with recitations of Kaddish (Rich, 1996).

Throughout the formal mourning period as well as annual memorial observances of the deceased, reciting Kaddish is an integral and extremely important component of the grieving and remembering process. This version of the Kaddish is supplied by Rich (1996).

Mourner's Kaddish

> ''May His great Name grow exalted and sanctified (Cong. Amen.)
> in the world that He created as He willed.
> May He give reign to His Kingship in your lifetimes and in your days,
> and in the lifetimes of the entire Family of Israel,
> swiftly and soon, Now respond: Amen.
> (Cong. Amen. May His great Name be blessed forever and ever.)
> May His great Name be blessed forever and ever.
> Blessed, praised, glorified, exalted, extolled,
> mighty, upraised, and lauded be the name of the Holy One, Blessed is He
> (Cong. Blessed is He) beyond any blessing and song,
> praise and consolation that are uttered in the world. Now respond: Amen.
> (Cong. Amen.)
> He who makes peace in His heights, may He make peace,
> upon us and upon all Israel. Now respond: Amen.
> (Cong. Amen.)''

Concerning issues of providing spiritual care in a healthcare facility or some other institutional setting, nurses, chaplains, and any other individuals attempting to provide care should be mindful of the following things which are traditional concepts in Judaism (although there are exceptions):

- Illness is considered a community event; visiting the sick is a high priority.
- Do not expect all Jewish patients to have the same needs and beliefs; ask about beliefs and practices that may affect their hospital stay.
- Ask if patients would like to see a rabbi.
- Be aware that some religious artwork and symbols might be offensive.
- Do not refer to synagogue as "church."
- Be cognizant of appropriate and inappropriate holiday greetings.
- Be aware that some Jewish patients observe kosher dietary laws.
- Be aware of potential conflicts on end-of-life decisions:
  - obligation to heal
  - life to be preserved
  - death not to be prolonged
  - differences on these issues among various sects.
- Be aware of conflicting positions of various sects on life support:
  - Orthodox—life is sacred and to be preserved
  - Conservative and Reform—can let nature take its course in an irreversible, terminal illness situation
  - overall ambiguity between obligation to cure versus letting natural death occur.
- The body of the deceased is to be treated with utmost respect (very pronounced in Judaism because of its intense valuation of life).
- The body of the deceased is not to be left alone because it is considered disrespectful (i.e. family members will want to stay with the body until it is transported to the mortuary).

Furthermore, there are prayers (which are in fact Holy Scripture) that can be offered when a patient is approaching death or already dead.

Shema

> *"Hear O Israel, the Lord is our God, the Lord is One.*
> *May His name of glory and majesty be blessed forever.*
> *You shall love the Lord your God with all your heart, with all your soul, and in all your ways. These words that I am commanding you today shall be in your heart. You should teach them to your children, speak them while returning home, while traveling on your way, and while dwelling in your place. You shall tie them as a sign upon your hand, and as frontlets between your eyes. You should write them upon the doorposts of your house and gates."*

A Psalm of David

> *"The Lord is my shepherd; I shall not want.*
> *He maketh me to lie down in green pastures; He leadeth me beside the still waters.*
> *He restoreth my soul; He leadeth me in the paths of righteousness for His name's sake.*
> *Yea, though I walk through the valley of the shadow of death, I will fear no evil for Thou art with me; Thy rod and Thy staff they comfort me.*
> *Thou preparest a table before me in the presence of mine enemies;*
> *Thou annointest my head with oil; my cup runneth over.*
> *Surely, goodness and mercy shall follow me all the days of my life,*
> *and I will dwell in the house of the Lord forever."*

Finally, there are several things of which a guest should be aware when visiting a mourner (Kreindler, 2000; Rich, 1996):

- Do not attempt to express grief with standard, shallow platitudes.
- Do allow the mourner to initiate conversations.
- Do not redirect the conversation from talk about the deceased.
- Do encourage conversation about the deceased to help insure the full expression of grief.
- Do understand that the expressions of feeling towards God in distressful times are not heresy or lack of faith, but rather a struggle for faith.
- Do remember that it is traditional for a guest to say to mourners upon leaving their house the following:

> *"May the Lord comfort you with all the mourners of Zion and Jerusalem."*
> *Shalom!*

Native American

> *Aho, mitakuye oyasin!*
> *Aho, all my relations!*

According to Reverend Doctor Kara Hawkins (2000) of Spiritual Warrior Ministries, this Lakota phrase is reflective of an intrinsic Native American cultural view and understanding of one's relationship with the universe. This can be even better understood through the knowledge of the basic tenets of Native American philosophy:

- All is sacred.
- All is related.
- All is interconnected to the Great Web of Life.
- All is part of God, and God is immanent within all.

> *"As children of the One Father, Great Spirit, we are all relatives. Like an interwoven fabric, we are connected to all creation, and as such, what hurts one, hurts all; what honors one, honors all. We are connected in life and we are connected in death. We are in relation, therefore, to all things, all beings, all situations."*

This concept of existence, referred to as the Circle of Life or the Medicine Wheel (provided at the end of this section), is the Native American way of acknowledging, understanding, and experiencing one's relationship with the universe through the natural cycles of life: birth, maturation, transition, death, rebirth. Concerning these, Hawkins (2000) says the following:

> *"We experience these cycles in the changing of the seasons, as we move from sunrise to sunrise, and as we sow our seeds and reap what we sow."*
>
> *Hawkins (2000)*

She further notes that the Native American's circular, holistic understanding of life and death is different from Western civilization's more linear and compartmentalized perspective of life. This supports the concept that Native Americans are more right-brain oriented than they are left-brain oriented: Right brain being *affective* and left brain being *cognitive*. Thus, according to Hawkins (2000), Native Americans are keenly interested in the following:

- music
- color
- storytelling
- mind/body/spirit
- sound
- ritual/ceremony
- cosmology
- relationships.

These concepts are reflected, especially that of relationships, in the 12-fold "Traditional Indian Code of Ethics."

1. Give thanks to the Creator each morning upon rising and each evening before sleeping. Seek courage to be a better person.
2. Showing respect is a basic law of life.
3. Respect the wisdom of people in council. Once you give an idea it no longer belongs to you.
4. Be truthful at all times.
5. Always treat your guests with honor and consideration. Give your best food and comforts to your guests.
6. The hurt of one is the hurt of all. The honor of one is the honor of all.
7. Receive strangers and outsiders kindly.
8. All races are children of the Creator and must be respected.

9. To serve others, to be of some use to family, community, or nation is one of the main purposes for which people are created. True happiness comes to those who dedicate their lives to the service of others.
10. Observe moderation and balance in all things.
11. Know those things that lead to your well-being and those things that lead to your destruction.
12. Listen and follow the guidance given to your heart. Expect guidance to come in many forms: in prayer, in dreams, in solitude and in the words and actions of elders and friends.

With respect to death, it is but one turn on the Medicine Wheel as a time for rest and renewal, a time to prepare for rebirth. Rebirth for the Native American holds many interpretations and understandings depending upon tribal orientation and religious beliefs. Some of these include Christianity's understanding of rebirth into the hereafter (i.e. heaven or the Spirit World). Other beliefs include reincarnation on the earth plane or journeying to another stellar system.

For families and loved ones observing native customs, Hawkins stresses that the time of their loved one's transition into the Spirit World is a critical one and that there are certain customs observed for protection of the deceased's family and friends. One such custom is to refrain from speaking the deceased's name aloud. It is believed that to do so might draw the attention of the deceased's Spirit back to the earth plane, perhaps slow its progress to the Spirit World or possibly adversely affect the living. This effect might take the form of illness in the deceased's family. When referring to the deceased, therefore, you would instead refer to his or her relation to the individual you are addressing (e.g., ''your father,'' ''your mother,'' ''your friend,'' etc).

Furthermore, in times of serious illness, death and dying, ceremony and ritual (highly personal and family oriented) are necessary and critical for preparing the patient and his or her relatives for the transition to the next life. Therefore, prior to meeting with the dying or deceased person's family and friends, it would be helpful for the pastoral care giver to find out what the facility's rules are concerning the practice of religious rituals. The purpose of ceremony and ritual is to bring the patient's and family's consciousness into the present moment's awareness so that healing can take place on all levels—mind, body, spirit. Moreover, sound, color, touch, movement, aromatherapy used in ceremony and ritual move one's consciousness to an altered state wherein one may access the Collective Conscious-Higher Self-God. Important rituals are the following:

- incense burning, such as is used by the Native Americans
- singing of ceremonial song accompanied by drum or rattle
- smoking of the Sacred Pipe.

The Burning of Sage, Sweet-grass and/or Cedar Incense

In Native American Spirituality, a common practice for purification and preparation of oneself and one's space for ceremony is the burning of the sacred herbs of sage and/or cedar, sweet-grass or tobacco. Often placed in an abalone shell or other natural container, the sacred smoke is fanned to the West, North, East, South, to the Heavens above and to the Earth below, praying to Great Spirit for purification, protection, and guidance for all those present and for all their relations. (Note:

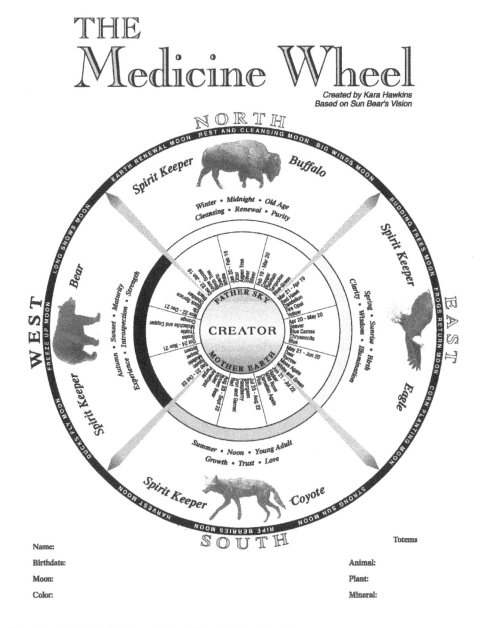

THE
Medicine Wheel

Created by Kara Hawkins
Based on Sun Bear's Vision

Name:

Birthdate:

Moon:

Color:

Totems

Animal:

Plant:

Mineral:

Reproduced with the kind permission of Rev. Dr. Kara Hawkins.

because the smell of burning sage can sometimes be mistaken for marijuana, the care givers and the healthcare facility's administration need clarification concerning the distinction.)

Ceremonial Song Accompanied by Drum or Rattle

One form this prayer may take is the Four Directions Song. According to Hawkins (2000), the drum and rattle, far more than just accompaniment to the ceremonial song, calls forth the Spirits of the Grandfathers, Father Sky and Mother Earth, so that people may enter into sacred awareness of their relation to Great Spirit, their Grandfather, who is everywhere: Above, below, to the right and left, before and behind. The singer, offering a pinch of tobacco or fanning the smoke of the sacred herbs to each direction, sings (loosely translated to English):

> *''Look towards the West! Your Grandfather is sitting there looking this way.*
> *Pray to Him! Pray to Him!*
> *He is sitting there looking this way.*
>
> *Look towards the North! Your Grandfather is sitting there looking this way.*
> *Pray to Him! Pray to Him!*
> *He is sitting there looking this way.*
>
> *Look towards the East! Your Grandfather is sitting there looking this way.*
> *Pray to Him! Pray to Him!*
> *He is sitting there looking this way.*
>
> *Look towards the South! Your Grandfather is sitting there looking this way.*
> *Pray to Him! Pray to Him!*
> *He is sitting there looking this way.*
>
> *Look up above! The Great Spirit. He is sitting above us.*
> *Pray to Him! Pray to Him!*
> *He is sitting there looking this way.*
>
> *Look down at the Earth! Your Grandmother is lying beneath you.*
> *Pray to Her! Pray to Her!*
> *She is lying there listening to your prayers.''*

Singer and teacher of ceremonial song and drum for the last 20 years, Hawkins (2000) says that all vibration is Spirit and that the most sacred and healing of instruments is the voice. One can readily see, then, because of this belief, the importance of song and drum in the healing and prayer rituals for the sick and dying.

Smoking of the Sacred Pipe

For many practitioners of Native American Spirituality, praying with the Sacred Pipe is central to their faith. A highly personal ritual, prayers are made in the form of pinches of pure tobacco or natural blending of herbs (no drugs are ever used) and offered to the Four Directions and Father Sky and Mother Earth. After this, those prayers, in the tangible form of tobacco, are placed in the bowl of the pipe. The Pipe Filling Ritual is usually accompanied by song. As the pipe is lit, it is first offered to the Grandfathers "so that they may 'smoke' first." The pipe is then passed in a clockwise manner for all to share. When sharing the Sacred Pipe, the pipe bowl is accepted in the left hand, stem in the right. It is smoked without inhaling, usually about four puffs. The smoke is drawn in lightly and released as "prayers made visible." The pipe is then turned ritually in a clockwise manner so as to honor the Grandfathers and passed to the left.

If the institution in which the Native American resides does not allow the burning of incense or tobacco, Hawkins (2000) suggests that since intent is most important, the rituals may still be practiced without the burning. The sage bowl, for example, may be ritually fanned to the Grandfathers and the filled pipe may be ritually passed for others to pray over without burning. For many practitioners, this "spiritual smoking" is no less an effective prayer. The pipe holder would then smoke the prayers at a later time.

Another ritual, "Keeping of the Soul," is observed in many ways. For one, an individual authorized by the family as the Soul's Keeper (i.e. keeper of the Spirit of the deceased) might clip a lock of the deceased's hair as a part of the keeping, praying over and caring for the Soul. At the first-year anniversary of the person's death, a family memorial service is conducted in which the soul is ritually released.

Memorial services for the deceased Native American may take many forms. Hawkins (2000) explains that since Native American Spirituality is a way of life rather than a religion, it is not uncommon for Native peoples to embrace both their Native faith traditions as well as the practice of another faith, such as Baha'i, Christianity, etc. Because of this fact, the faith needs of seriously ill and dying Native American patients must be investigated. Thus, the memorial service may be syncretistic or specifically Native American. Note these words of Hawkins (2000) as she describes what might be constituent elements of a typical Native American memorial service.

> *"Traditionally, depending on one's tribal orientations, the Sacred Pipe is prayed with, or pinches of tobacco are offered to the Spirits of the Four Directions with prayer or ceremonial song. The smoke of the sacred herbs is fanned ritually to the Spirits of the Directions, Father Sky and Mother Earth, often with an eagle's wing (by one authorized to have it) as it is believed the Spirit of the Eagle will take our prayers to the Creator."*
>
> *Hawkins (2000)*

Additionally, other elements of a memorial service are similar to those of other faith traditions: offering of prayers for the deceased; offering of support for the bereaved; and offering of thanksgiving for the many ways the deceased has blessed the lives of relatives and loved ones. However, ritual observances of the deceased do not end with the funeral services. For many Native Americans, a time of prayer and reflection on the first-year anniversary is observed. If there has been a "Soul Keeping Ritual," at this time the soul is released ritually. The family of the deceased, who have prepared all year for this time of release, hosts a memorial dinner that includes a giveaway for all who attend. A giveaway, traditional for most Native peoples, is a giving away (usually at much sacrifice for the host family) of blankets, household goods, and perhaps possessions of the deceased such as personal pipes and sacred objects. With this cultural view of Native American spirituality in mind, the pastoral care or healthcare provider can enter into a more helpful relationship with the family and friends of the deceased Native American.

With respect to organ and/or tissue donation, the decision is one of individual choice. The same is also true concerning embalming and disposition of the body: cremation or burial. Furthermore, when meeting with the bereaved family members, do not assume their religious orientation is exclusively Native American. Rather, it is best to ask politely to talk with the family group's representative spokesperson in order to determine their wishes for their deceased loved one.

Finally, when attempting to provide compassionate care to the bereaved the following suggestions should be considered:

- Be aware of the unique nature of Native American spirituality.
- Do not interrupt family members who are talking to each other. Wait until the conversation is concluded and they turn to you.
- If one is chosen to lead the service, accord that one the same respect you would a minister of any other religious tradition.
- Do not stare into the eyes of the one to whom you are speaking. Look away as much as you can while talking.
- Speak in soft, even tones.
- Offer your hand when introducing yourself to each member of the family or friends assembled, then again when you are leaving. Be sure that your grip is not a hard one.
- If the family does not have anyone present to lead in ceremony and ritual, do not attempt to perform any of the rituals previously described, unless they are of your own spiritual practice.
- Pray as you would in your own tradition using language widely accepted among faith traditions (e.g. ''O Creator ...'' or ''O God ...''). Then ask if someone else present has a prayer to offer. If not, Hawkins (2000) suggests the following:

> ''All My Relations, Grandfather, Grandmother, hear our Prayers for [remember not to say the name of the deceased; but refer to relationship; e.g. this loved one, son and grandson]. Bless him [or her] O Grandfather and guide his [her] Spirit as only you know, Grandfather. Bless all of us here and help us with our sadness, O Grandfather, that we may not cause the Spirit of our Loved One to look back upon us. Keep us safe, O Grandfather, and guide us and all our loved ones so that we may live in a good way for all our relations.
> Beauty before me,
> Beauty behind me
> Beauty to the left of me and Beauty to the right of me
> Beauty above me and Beauty below me
> I walk in Beauty, In Beauty I walk.
>
> Spirit before you,
> Spirit behind you
> Spirit to the left of you and Spirit to the right of you
> Spirit above you and Spirit below you
> You walk in Spirit, In Spirit you walk.
>
> Beauty before us,
> Beauty behind us
> Beauty to the left of us and Beauty to the right of us.
> Beauty above us and Beauty below us
> We walk in Beauty, In Beauty we walk.
>
> Aho, mitakuye oyasin [pronounced, Ah ho meetakwe yahsee].
> All my relations.''

13

What About Final Arrangements?

> *"Everyone knows they're going to die, but nobody believes it. If we did, we would do things differently."*
>
> Morrie Schwartz in *Tuesdays with Morrie (Albom, 1997, p. 81)*

Since death is final, it is reasonable to say that arrangements concerning a deceased individual would be classified as final: burial, cremation, embalming, cemetery, funeral/memorial service, etc. When, though, should such arrangements be made and by whom? It is precisely those and other questions which we will address in this chapter.

In an article entitled "What Families Should Know About Funeral-Related Costs: Implications for Social Work Practice," Mercedes Bern-Klug *et al.* identify seven factors that contribute to the uniqueness of making final arrangements (1999, pp. 128–137):

1. The person or people responsible for making funeral arrangements or overseeing the implementation of preneed arrangements are typically in crisis and over-whelmed by grief.
2. Final arrangements can be expensive: the most expensive purchase many people will make, behind the cost of a house, a car and a wedding.
3. The finality of the decisions contributes to the uniqueness of making the arrange-ments: no returns, exchanges, or cash refunds.
4. People are often pressed for time when it comes to making final arrangements: usually within 24 hours after the death.
5. Confusion about the primary purpose of the funeral may exist:
   - providing public recognition that a death has occurred
   - providing a framework in which to support those most affected by the death
   - providing a means of disposing of the deceased's body
   - providing a way to honor the life of the deceased
   - providing a way of recognizing the reality and finality of death and aiding in "integration of the loss."
6. The person purchasing the goods and services is grossly inexperienced in making such a costly purchase with so many options offered.
7. There seems to be a lack of clarity in our society about the etiquette and protocol of final arrangements.
   - Should one compare funeral costs among those who offer these services?
   - Should one negotiate prices over goods and services with a funeral director?

Not only do these and other factors contribute to the uniqueness of making final arrangements, they also heighten an already stressful time.

In an extremely useful booklet, *Funeral Related Options and Costs: A Guide for Families* (1996), Bern-Klug masterfully and succinctly addresses many of those factors as well as the questions posed in the first paragraph: the "when" and "who" concerning final arrangements. Much of what follows is excerpted from that booklet, which we highly recommend.

Decisions about final arrangements are personal, emotional, and can be meaningful. They can also be costly; price ranges for the "same" services vary, sometimes greatly. This word of counsel is in order if pre-arrangement has not occurred.

> *"Do not let emotions or the closeness of the relationship to the deceased be the determining factors in how much money to spend on the various components of final arrangements. On the contrary, let reason and economic prudence guide the decision-making process."*
>
> *SLJ*

What does it mean to pre-arrange, preplan final arrangements? Do such terms mean that everything, including payment of all expenses, is taken care of prior to the death? The answer to the latter question is "yes" and "no." Those "pre" words can be comprehensive and inclusive of the vast majority of things associated with final arrangements, including payment. (The one possible exception to a prepaid expense would be to the cemetery for the "opening and closing of the grave.") The nomenclature utilized in the funeral professions for this type of arrangement (i.e. monetary) is "preneed." On the other hand, those "pre" words can mean the communication of one's wishes in writing or verbally concerning final arrangements before death, without prepayment.

> *"It is always appropriate to pre-plan (discuss); but be careful how you pre-pay."*
> *Mercedes Bern-Klug (1996)*

Concerning preneed plans (those which include prepayment) Bern-Klug (1996) states that there are several important things to consider (i.e. a clear understanding of answers to pertinent questions) before purchase and subsequent payment:

- What happens to the money I prepay? Make certain you get official documentation of where the funds are deposited.
- How much time do I have to reconsider my purchase and receive a full refund?
- What happens to my money if the funeral home is purchased by another funeral home or goes out of business?
- What happens if I die away from home?
- Even if I prepurchase this funeral plan, what expenses will my survivors have to pay later? What is *not* covered?
- Am I prepaying for specific items that the funeral home or cemetery will store until needed (e.g. casket, vault, etc.) or will my survivors choose the casket or vault based on what is available at the time of need?

The answers to these questions can be very helpful to and less stressful for survivors. Note the data in Table 13.1 compiled by Bern-Klug (1996) from the Funeral Information Project she directed in 1995.

Table 13.1   Is making funeral arrangements before death helpful to survivors?

No	9%
Somewhat	24%
Extremely helpful	67%

A very detailed discussion of final arrangement costs and preneed arrangement options is found on pages 3–7 and a sample "General Price List" is found on pages 13–15 of the booklet written by Bern-Klug (1996).

If no prearrangement dialogue has occurred or a preneed plan has not been purchased, Bern-Klug (1996) identifies four key decisions the survivors must make following a death:

- Decide on what to do with the body.
- Decide on goods and services to be purchased.
- Decide on ceremony to acknowledge the death and/or celebrate the life.
- Decide on ideas for "memorializing" the life following the ceremony.

Additionally, it is prudent to decide on ideas for how these issues will be handled.

- **What to do with the body**: There are four options to consider:
  1. earth burial
  2. entombment above ground in a mausoleum
  3. cremation
  4. donation of body for scientific research.
- **Goods and services to be purchased**: The goods and services most generally are obtained from three sources—the funeral home, the cemetery, and the florist. (The following discussion addresses only the first two.)
  1. The funeral home: From the funeral home, one can purchase the casket or urn and make arrangements for the funeral or memorial service. Prices for these goods and services vary greatly. Because of that fact, it is important to remember this insight from Bern-Klug:

  > *"The cost of a funeral is not related to its meaningfulness."*
  >
  > *Bern-Klug (1996)*

At the same time, it is also important to give serious consideration to the suggestions and options offered by the funeral director. The vast majority of people in the funeral profession are courteous, respectful, and sensitive to the needs of people at this very difficult time in their lives. Such is confirmed by the results of Bern-Klug's Funeral Information Project (*see* Table 13.2).

Table 13.2 "At the funeral home, how well did the staff treat the family (were you treated with respect, dignity, and concern)?"

Treated very well	94%
Treated okay	5%
Treated poorly	1%

2. **The cemetery:** The services provided by the cemetery are typically called the "opening and closing of the grave" for earth burials. If you have a preneed plan, the charge for this service is generally not included. The goods one usually purchases from a cemetery, depending on the type of disposition, are as follows:
   - grave plot
   - crypt space in a mausoleum
   - cremation box or urn

- niche in a columbarium
- burial containers for caskets, of which there are two types:
  a. grave liners—not sealed (does not protect casket)
  b. vaults—sealed (does protect casket)
- grave markers, of which there are two types:
  a. monuments—upright
  b. grass marker—lays flat against the ground.
- **Ceremony to acknowledge the death and/or celebrate the life**: Funeral or memorial services, commonly preceded by the wake or visitation, take place in any number of places:
  - funeral home
  - faith community place of worship
  - cemetery chapel and/or graveside
  - home of the deceased, family member, or friend
  - park or garden area,
- The funeral/memorial service is a very beneficial and yet difficult time for survivors of the deceased. How important is the support of others for the deceased's immediate family? One Funeral Information Project respondent comments:

  "Family and friends are so important during the funeral services and after. It's a very difficult time. Friends need to remember their support and love are needed for months after the funeral. It's so hard getting over the loss."

- **Memorializing the life following the ceremony**: Keeping the memory alive by honoring the life can be expensive or cost very little. The following is a list of ideas:
  - Write a detailed obituary.
  - Write a detailed funeral program, including photographs.
  - Write a short story of cherished memories of the deceased and share it with family and friends.
  - Establish a scholarship at a school, college, faith congregation, hospital, etc. in the name of the deceased.
  - Plant a tree or some type of shrubbery/flowering bush in some special place.
  - Donate money or items to charity in the name of the deceased.
  - Put up a plaque in a public or private place with the name, picture, and/or some saying about the deceased inscribed thereon.
  - Keep pictures out and up in the house or carry pictures with you.
  - Name the name on a regular basis in conversation with people.

  "A loved one is not 'gone' until two things happen—we stop saying the name and we begin editing this individual out of our stories."

  HIS

Concerning who makes and/or should make final arrangements, survey responses from 163 survivors of older adults in Kansas City showed that adult children play an important role in the final arrangements of a parent, either as the key arranger or the primary one who accompanies the surviving parent or spouse (given the number of non-first marriages). Fifty percent of those responsible for making final arrangements had no idea what to expect in terms of cost. Furthermore, my (SLJ) experience in ministry with grieving families in the hospital is that a goodly number of adult children or surviving spouses respond with "What do we do now?" when their loved one takes the last breath. Much of this additional anxiety in an already anxiety-intense atmosphere could be alleviated through conversations with family members and careful preplanning. When should preplanning occur? One participant in the funeral study relates:

> *"The best time to discuss final arrangements was at a family picnic 'with the sun shining and everybody healthy' ... once serious illness strikes, it may be too painful to discuss."*

I (SLJ) do not know that a family picnic is the ideal setting for such a discussion, but consider these words:

> *"Pre-planning, at the very least, when one is healthy and young minimizes the trauma of death for the survivors."*
>
> *SLJ*

How does one begin the process of preplanning final arrangements? Start with a family discussion. You might also want to talk with friends who have recently experienced the death of a loved one. It could be prudent to involve a clergy person or individual you desire to perform the funeral/memorial service in the discussion in order to receive more objective input. Finally, learn about the options and costs associated with them from conversations with funeral directors and from materials such as *Funeral Related Options and Costs: A Guide for Families* (Bern-Klug 1996) and resources provided by AARP.

Increasingly, people are visiting funeral home web sites before calling a funeral director. Five items to consider before talking to a funeral director are the following:

1. What is the estimated budget for final arrangements?
2. How should the costs be paid?
3. How will this question be answered: "How would you like to handle these expenses?"
4. How much of the life insurance proceeds should be spent on final arrangements?
5. Where are the documents needed to make the arrangements?

The funeral director can be helpful with some of these questions, but you and you alone should determine how much you can afford to spend. Many survivors have struggled financially following the death of a loved one because they spent more than they could afford on the loved one's funeral.

> *"Living within your means includes expenses associated with final arrangements for a loved one."*
>
> *SLJ*

In a presentation entitled "Planning the Gift of Love" that I (SLJ) make on a regular basis in faith congregations, businesses and schools, concerning the necessity of preplanning one's healthcare, one slide reads as shown in Box 13.1.

Box 13.1

Your ''Gift of Love'' basket should include:

Savings	Investment planning
Income protection	Retirement planning
(i.e. insurance)	
Debt management	Healthcare planning
Education planning	Estate planning

Perhaps one additional item should be added: ''Final Arrangements Planning.'' It should include ideas relevant to each of the five key decisions following a death that must be made:

1. What to do with the body.
2. What goods and services are to be purchased.
3. What type of ceremony to have.
4. What and how to memorialize the life.
5. How these issues will be handled.

One would also need to know how to pay for all of the things associated with those arrangements. Will it be personal savings, life insurance, some preneed plan purchased from a funeral home? Thoughtful contemplation of those issues in the same manner as planning for the education of your children, retirement, and the disposition of your estate at death would be prudent.

   Unfortunately, the ideal is not always the reality. Nevertheless, it is a worthy goal. In conclusion, the overarching purpose of this chapter is to raise the awareness of professional and lay care givers of the advantages of planning final arrangements before the death and, thus, make them proactive advocates for the implementation of such. Where can this take place? In faith congregations and educational forums in a variety of other venues: civic clubs, ''Lunch and Learn'' events in the workplace, community-focused programs through academic institutions. Resources for such instructional programs can be hospital chaplains, social workers (especially those who work with Hospice), financial planners, and funeral directors.

   > ''One of the greatest gifts you can bestow on family and loved ones is to preplan your healthcare, prepare an estate document, preplan final arrangements, and make certain someone knows the location of key documents.''
   >
   > SLJ

To obtain a copy of the book, *Funeral Related Options and Costs: A Guide for Families* (Bern-Klug, 1996), address correspondence to:

Center on Aging/FIP
University of Kansas Medical Center
5026 Wescoe
Kansas City
KS 66160–7117

14

Rituals: A Necessity For Healthy Grief

I (HIS) contend that rituals give an individual a "corporate" way to acknowledge the death (Harold Ivan Smith, 2001, p. 56):

- Rituals help survivors publicly acknowledge the reality of the loss.
- Rituals acknowledge friends' and neighbors' grief.
- Rituals provide a venue to celebrate the life of the deceased.
- Rituals provide a way to corporately express good-byes.
- Rituals provide a way to offer support to the chief mourners.
- Rituals provide ways to promise future support and care.
- Rituals give an opportunity to be with others who, too, have lost.

Rabbi Michael Zedek (1999) suggested that rituals are tripartite in meaning with the goal of *"requiring us to act our way into right thinking:"*

1. to help us acknowledge what has happened
2. to help us know what we are when something has happened
3. to help us proceed when something has happened.

Through planning, preparing, and implementing rituals in concert with grievers, pastoral care givers facilitate "making special." Kim Logan of Kansas City Hospice and Harold Ivan Smith say that a meaningful ritual can be created by following certain steps:

- Evaluate former rituals: Did they "work?" How might they be improved? (Smith)
- Solicit information from other ritual leaders. Their discoveries or innovations could enhance the quality of your ritual. (Smith)
- Focus on a goal. What is the desired outcome for the ritual? (Logan)
- Plan. Let ideas flow and pick and choose among them. (Logan)
- Flesh out details before making a final choice. (Logan)
- Prepare. Gather the materials and resources that will be needed. (Logan)
- Incorporate the ritual into your memory. (Logan)

> *"Rituals are a bridge between the world in which the loved one existed and the emerging world without the deceased."*
>
> HIS

Historically, family and close friends were expected to attend all three rituals associated with death:

1. visitation/wake
2. funeral/memorial service
3. committal.

In the following pages, we will discuss these rituals along with variations of them and conclude with some words for pastoral care givers.

The Visitation/Wake

No one should have to go through bereavement alone, particularly initial bereavement. That concept is universal among all people. Because of this fact, rituals are a vital necessity for grievers. The first of the rituals is the viewing of the deceased, more commonly known as the visitation or wake. Alan Wolfelt relates how important this ritual is:

> *"For mourners, an invitation to see the body is an invitation to say goodbye and to touch someone they love for the last time. It is also an invitation to confront their disbelief that someone they deeply cared for is gone and cannot return. Far from being morbid, open caskets help acknowledge the reality of death and the transition from life before the loss to life after."*
>
> *Alan Wolfelt (1997a, p. 20)*

Thus, the visitation is an important ritual of leave taking. It helps in those first hours of what Johnson calls *"the great darkness of grief"* (1999, p. 9). The stories, the hugs, faces, tears of friends and neighbors communicate: "You are not alone in this; you will not be abandoned." The visitation offers an opportunity for people to communally confront the reality of this particular death. Although details vary, this concept of companioning through the rituals is an integral part of all religious traditions.

> *"The time immediately following death is often one of bewilderment and may involve shock or heart-rending grief for the family and close friends ... ministry at this time is one of gently accompanying the mourners in their initial adjustment to the fact of death and the sorrow this entails."*
>
> *The International Commission on English in the Liturgy, 1990, p. 21*

However, the visitation is not only important for those who go through the journey of rituals with the family, but also for:

- those who cannot attend the funeral service because of work, other commitments, or time constraints
- those who are uncomfortable in or do not like crowds
- those who dislike, for whatever reasons, funeral services
- those who have had recent or negative funeral experiences.

Moreover, in this busy society, time off from work or being away from other commitments is not easily arranged for multiple rituals. Therefore, some families fear that if they have rituals on separate days, few will attend. One response to that dilemma is to combine the viewing and the memorial service so that the visitation takes place immediately prior to the funeral service.

As pastoral care givers, it is important to communicate to grievers that visitations have a vital but informal role to play in ritualizing the dead. I (HIS) was reconvinced of the value of the visitation when my mother died. I was surprised by the turnout of people and how thoroughly I enjoyed the chance to visit with old friends, extended family members, and neighbors. I (SLJ) have the same sentiment as well. At my father's visitation, I saw people I had not seen in years. The time we spent together was very meaningful. Given the mobility of our society, the visitation plays an important role in the rekindling of previous relationships. Moreover, the visitation is not as impacted by time schedule as a funeral/committal.

Obviously, visitation practices vary in different locales. A specific local custom is best learned by talking with local clergy and/or funeral directors.

The Funeral/Memorial Service

Why have a funeral? More and more people these days are asking that question. Alan Wolfelt offers some insight into this mindset:

> *"For many, traditional funeral rituals have lost much of their value and meaning. They are perceived as empty and lacking creativity. I myself have attended way too many of what I would term cookie-cutter ceremonies that leave you feeling like you may as well have been at a stranger's funeral. As more and more people attend these meaningless funerals, society's opinion of the funeral ritual nosedives."*
>
> *Alan Wolfelt (1994, p. 7)*

Furthermore, in a culture that values convenience and efficiency, there has been a startling increase in what is termed "direct disposal," which translates as no viewing, no services, and immediate cremation—a reality I (HIS) experienced when my uncle died. Even if there is a service, it is very brief with "family only" graveside services or scattering of the ashes. It is not unusual to read in newspaper obituaries: *"At the request of the deceased, no visitation or services have been scheduled."*

In response to this trend, some funeral directors, pastoral care givers and clinicians have found that a number of those who chose direct disposal have experienced difficulty reconciling with the death. One funeral director relates this story of a family who wanted direct disposal when their mother died. There was no visitation, no funeral service, no burial, not even a formal scattering of the ashes. A year later when the father died, the funeral director was approached by the family: "Mom's funeral (really nonfuneral) wasn't right. What shall we do?" The funeral director suggested a traditional funeral, and the family agreed. However, an interesting thing happened at the committal. A grandson asked, "Okay, I see where Grandpa is; now, where is Grandma?" Here, it took a nine-year-old boy to educate adults of the value of a traditional funeral (McCormick, 2000, May, p. 23).

James F. White (1990) offers two arguments against direct disposals. He relates that funeral rituals accomplish the following:

1. console the bereaved
2. formally commend the deceased to God.

Wolfelt (1997b) identifies these functions for a funeral today:

1. Helps us acknowledge that someone we love has died.
2. Allows us to say goodbye.
3. Helps us remember the person who died and encourages us to share those memories with others.
4. Affirms the worth of our relationship with the person who died.
5. Provides a social support system for us and for other friends and family members.
6. Allows us to search for meaning of life and death.
7. Offers continuity and a hope for the living (p. 32).

Additionally, a funeral provides a model or point of reference for future funeral services.

I (HIS) find a societal need for a funeral ritual.

"A time for a pause in the rhythm of life to say a public good-bye."

HIS

So, if there is to be a public service, should the body of the deceased or the cremated human remains be present? The reality is that memorial services without the body are an alternative preferred by many families. There are at least two factors that make this attractive:

1. **Timing and convenience**: With no body to be buried and the ritual not being governed by transportation factors or regular cemetery hours, services can be scheduled days, weeks, even months after the death. Furthermore, the services can be scheduled in late afternoon, early evening, or on weekends, more convenient times for potential attendees.
2. **Cost**: A memorial service, particularly coupled with cremation, is a way significantly to reduce costs. In reality, money influences many ritual choices, especially when there is tension among family members or when there are limited financial resources to cover expenses.

Alan Wolfelt insists that this abbreviated, bare minimum type of memorial service tends to encourage mourners to skirt the healing potential of the pain. In fact, he laments: *"How many times have you heard someone leave a memorial service saying, 'Wasn't that great? No one even cried!'"* He adds, *"while some memorial services are certainly meaningful and authentic, I am suggesting that too often they do healthy mourning a disservice"* (1994, pp. 8–9).

Joseph Bankoff describes his neighbor's funeral:

"We buried my neighbor Bob Strickland this week.

We celebrated seven decades of his achievements ending in several years of grace as he fought his last battle with his own body ... They did not talk about his accomplishments. We knew them well. Instead, we were reminded of the encouragement that Bob Strickland gave to everyone around him ... 'Howdy neighbor. I'm sure glad to see you.'"

Joseph Bankoff (1994, p. D9)

Why has there been a marked shift in the way Americans ritualize their dead? The answer is that we are a nomadic society. One in five Americans will move in a given year. After arriving at their new home, many will conclude: "Why bother to put down roots; who knows how long we will be here?" Because of this, neighbor and friend are not necessarily synonyms in today's society.

Unfortunately Walfoort is accurate in his assessment of American culture (1998, November 27, p. A5):

"Americans trade friends, familiarity and a larger yard for a bigger house, a better salary and the opportunities afforded by a larger city."

Increasingly through a series of relocations, corporate employees have lost a strong community of support. Furthermore, travel is a component of many people's jobs. Therefore, after a funeral, people leave the immediate family to "go to work" hundreds of miles away for days, weeks, or even months at a time. Consequently, there is no time for the traditional ritualizing and mourning thereafter.

This mobility of society, among other reasons, has increasingly caused families to choose no traditional ritual. This is especially true when family members insist, "He wasn't very religious." Alternatively, people elect for a "tribute" to the deceased or the "gathering" as an informal reception. Furthermore, after a year-long study of funeral rituals, Thomas G. Long concludes:

> *"If present trends continue, funeral directors and clergy can expect an increase in the pressure to become 'interior decorators of ritual,' designing environments, ad hoc services, and individualized occasions that suit this or that whim."*
>
> *Thomas G. Long (1997, p. 16)*

Moreover, according to William Aaron (former president of the National Funeral Directors Association), "For the first time in history, we are confronted with a 'death-free' generation—a generation where many have never experienced the loss of a loved one, or, for that matter, even attended a funeral" (2000, p. 4). So, when death comes, there has been no model of a "traditional" ritual to follow. Simplicity, creativity and innovation serve the moment. Aaron summarizes the forthcoming changes in the funeral industry:

> *"We can expect the face of the funeral service to change in just about every aspect ... The answer to the future is that we must adjust and change our business practices to meet the needs of client families in the new millennium."*
>
> *William Aaron (1999, p. 5)*

Are Aaron's words true? Unfortunately, they are true in some communities and rapidly expanding to others. However, the same is, also, true in other service-oriented professions. Years ago, not only did people know the local funeral director, but the banker, the pharmacist, the grocery store owner as well. Now, many of the "home-owned" business entities have been subsumed under a corporate umbrella complete with new management personnel. Excellent service, though, can be and is still available. Nevertheless, things are different and disconcerting to many.

> *"If leadership in pastoral care for the bereaved was ever needed, it is needed today."*
>
> *SLJ*

Another recent shift in the funeral ritual is its location. With the chapels in funeral homes, why take the additional time and create more expense by transferring the body to a church, synagogue, mosque, temple when the family only wants a brief, inexpensive service? Moreover, in urban settings the logistics of such a transfer, including a procession to the cemetery, can be a virtual nightmare, especially at or near "rush hour." Traffic flow may determine the length of the service. Robert Blair offers his assessment of this trend:

> *"I know of no spiritual reason why they (funerals) should be held in church sanctuaries, but I can think of many practical reasons for conducting them in mortuary chapels in urban areas ... The mortuary facilities are usually better suited for funeral arrangements ... However, it is good to accommodate any family that prefers to use the church building."*
>
> *Robert Blair (1998, p. 23)*

For some, the decision for the funeral chapel is based primarily on convenience and economy. For others, a psychological factor may influence the decision. For example, many individuals are told, "If you have the service for your loved one in a faith community facility, then every time you go there you will be reminded of your loss."

In response to this mindset, Wolfelt cries out that Americans "as a culture appear to be forgetting the importance of the funeral ritual" (1994, p. 5). "This society," he continues, "seems to be heading toward minimizing, avoiding, or denying the need for rituals surrounding death."

Thomas L. Long relates:

> *"Funerals were not merely 'nice things said about the deceased' but were religious dramas played out in the public theater of worship. Walking down the familiar and well-worn paths of the funeral was the community's way of reaffirming its faith—this is what we know, this is what we believe, this is how we shall live."*
>
> *Thomas L. Long (1997, p. 14)*

This assessment is characteristic of virtually every faith tradition. Funerals were once considered religious events governed by the liturgical style and tradition of a particular faith community. The same is still true today, although to a lesser degree in some traditions. Even when the deceased was not "religious," a clergy person was often summoned by the family or the funeral director to conduct the rituals. Long identifies three significant modern trends which challenge the traditional funeral:

1. movement from sacred space to "homelessness"
2. movement from sacred community to individualism
3. movement from sacred story to "personal best."

With respect to **sacred space**, faith was traditionally woven around three points of reference on the compass: the home, the place of worship, and the cemetery. Having this triad of sacred points made the decision of where to be ritualized and buried relatively easy. However, since people regularly move from place to place, putting down no roots in any one place, the decision of where to ritualize and bury is more complex. The move from sacred place has transformed many into spiritual nomads.

Concerning **sacred community**, it was not too many years ago that one's faith community was the center of one's life. This was especially true with the critically ill, dying and the bereaved. One of the first, if not *the* first, people summoned to the bedside of the sick or home of the bereaved was priest, pastor, rabbi, imam, etc. When my (SLJ) father died, I asked my mother whom she wanted called first. She responded: "the funeral home and the pastor." Not surprisingly, the visitation and funeral overflowed with people, not only from Dad's faith community, but the larger community as well. When Lloyd Jeffers died, the entire community grieved. To a certain extent, scenarios like this are still true in rural areas. However, in urban and suburban America, many people die outside of any faith or sense of larger community.

Regarding **sacred story**, the community once gathered for funerals to take solace in the "commonly held sacred story," which is different for the various religious traditions. But the things they all have in common are beliefs about life, death, after death (whether resurrection of the body, immortality of the soul, reincarnation). These elements were shared, sometimes through re-enactments, other times through various types of symbols. Increasingly, funerals today are moving away from sacred story to a celebration of the life of the deceased with very little, if any, religious addendum. Long critiques this contemporary trend in funerals:

> "In short, the commonly held sacred story gets lost amid a million-and-one 'me and my God' autobiographies. Thus, what may appear on the surface to be a refreshing and healthy trend in funerals—personalization, namely the amount of time and energy focused on the personality and life of the deceased—may in fact be a desperate attempt to fill the aching void left by the collapse of a creed we once believed in. When the larger story of God and humanity loses its power over our religious imaginations, then we are left to tell the only holy narrative we have left to tell—the biography of the deceased."
>
> Thomas L. Long (1997, p. 16)

Is it a case of either/or or both/and? Every person has his or her own opinion—although I (SLJ) would offer this suggestion for consideration. A balance between the celebration of the deceased's life and the telling of the sacred story (or how the sacred story was added to and played out in the deceased's life) seems to be a better way of helping a grieving family and loved ones move through those difficult days immediately following the death in a more healthy way. I base this assessment upon the funeral service of my dad, which was a blended service. Many people approached me at the cemetery, relating how meaningful the service was. There were also phone calls later that day and several days thereafter. In fact, my mother shared that people were talking about Dad's funeral for months.

Morrie Schwartz has some powerful words that give substance to the concepts of sacred space, sacred community, and sacred story:

> "The way you get meaning into your life is to devote yourself to loving others, devote yourself to the community around you, and devote yourself to creating something that gives you purpose and meaning."
>
> Morrie Schwartz (Albom, 1997, p. 43)

In conclusion, even though change is a constant with which we will continue to live (some of it bad, some of it good), pastoral care givers in concert with funeral directors can innovate and help to recreate sacred space, sacred community, and sacred story.

The Committal

The third component of ritualizing is the committal of the body or disposition of the cremated human remains. For some people, the committal is the most emotionally demanding component due to its sense of finality: the loved one will never be seen again. Because of this, there are people who attend the visitation and funeral, but will not go to the cemetery. Furthermore, some families make the decision for friends and loved ones not to go to the cemetery by selecting a family-only graveside service. Others indefinitely postpone scattering the ashes.

However, many grief specialists and funeral directors see the value of attending the committal. Thomas Lynch concurs:

"And you should see it till the very end. Avoid the temptation of a tidy leave taking in a room, a cemetery chapel, at the foot of the altar. None of that. Don't dodge it because of the weather. We've fished and watched football games in worse conditions. It won't take long. Go to the hole in the ground. Stand over it. Look into it. Wonder. And be cold. But stay until it's over. Until it is done."

Thomas Lynch (1997, p. 197)

Lynch is quite matter-of-fact in his counsel. Nevertheless, it is wise counsel. For many people, the time at the cemetery following the committal ceremony is very reminiscent of the visitation: socializing with family and friends whom you may not have seen in years and may not see again until another funeral or wedding. I (SLJ) have been to many committals and remember spending considerable time conversing with people who were not at the visitation. That very thing happened at my father's committal. It was good to see friends and family whom I had not seen for years. Unfortunately, living in a mobile society has a tendency to loosen close family/friend ties. A committal is an opportune moment to reconnect with and even rekindle those relationships that were once very special.

Moreover, time at the cemetery can be helpful in bringing closure. Jerry Kramer, a friend of the legendary football coach, Vince Lombardi, captures the finality:

"At the cemetery in New Jersey, I stood close to the coffin and kept waiting for something to happen. Now he's 'gonna' come out, I was thinking. Enough of this. I waited and waited, and the short ceremony was ended, and the family got up and left, and some guy next to me was clicking away with a camera, and I wanted to chew his head off, and all the people began to leave, and I waited, waited for something to happen, waited for someone to tell me the joke was over.

Soon some workmen came, and they put some dirty, ugly, rusty hooks on the four corners of the coffin, and they started to lower it into the ground. They got about halfway and I turned away. I couldn't watch it go down. I walked away. To me, he'll never be gone or buried."

Jerry Kramer (1970, p. 107)

The committal can be a meaningful time for those loved ones left behind. But is the committal only for the living? Consider the experience of a griever recounted by Harold Ivan Smith:

"It took me weeks last Fall to get over burying my friend Herb. I got soaked in the cold rain but it was my heart that hurt the most afterwards. But I do worry that when my time comes to ride in the hearse, no one will drive behind me on my last ride."

HIS (1996, p. 70)

So, the committal could equally be for the deceased, a way of showing that the life he or she lived did not go unnoticed. Understood in this way, then, the committal is a tribute to the deceased.

Finally, think long and hard before you decide not to attend the committal for a family member, loved one, or friend. You do not want to find yourself numbered among those who complain later that they felt cheated or deprived of the ritual, especially when they feel someone talked them out of it.

"I would rather regret having had a ritual than regret not having had one."

HIS

Concerns for Pastoral Care Givers

Bereavement is an invitation for pastoral care givers to be personally and significantly present. David Steere (2002) compared pastoral care to the tradition of sister-ships sent out to vessels in distress. The sister-ship comes alongside the damaged or idle ship, secures it with lines, and tows it to a safe harbor. In times of bereavement, pastoral care givers have the task of keeping grievers afloat and assist them to the safety of a harbor-like setting. Because of the importance of ritual for healthy grieving, harbor-like settings would include the visitation, the funeral, the committal, among other things.

The care giver's and funeral director's role in being those "sister-ships" is more important today than it was years ago, for according to Kenneth L. Woodward, an *"increasing number of Americans confront death with no inherited faith or liturgy for support"* (1998, p. 62). Therefore, their input is essential in helping to create sacred space, sacred community, and sacred story through those rituals surrounding death. Through such, families are better able to acknowledge and accept the reality of the loss and honor the life of the deceased.

Thus, pastoral care givers can partner with funeral directors to make certain that those final acts for the deceased are truly special for the family and other mourners. They have the opportunity to remind all who participate to do as Richard B. Gilbert suggests: *"Take off your shoes ... This is sacred ground"* (1998, p. 10).

Pastoral care givers must remember the importance of community as support for grievers, especially a faith community. These words of Kenneth Woodward are wise counsel:

> *"To die alone is bad enough, but to grieve without rituals that lift the broken heart is worse. Those whose grief is affirmed within a wider community of faith are fortunate."*
>
> *Kenneth Woodward (1998, p. 62)*

Rituals are an important mechanism for the larger community to express love to the deceased and the family. However, rituals should also include immediate family as recipients of not only the final act of love for the deceased but continuing love and support for them. As pastoral care givers, you can facilitate that happening.

Effective pastoral care is about:

- being interruptible to help a grieving family or friends plan for and carry out the rituals
- offering of presence in the lives of the grievers throughout the rituals
- waiting patiently with grievers, not dispensing easy answers
- listening to the losses of grievers
- being vulnerable
- being available after the rituals are concluded.

> *"Quality post-death rituals are important first steps in the journey of healthy grief."*
>
> *SLJ*

15

Concluding Words

I (SLJ) will never forget July 31, 1998. At 11:30 p.m. after a long journey, my wife, Jan, and I arrived in Okeechobee, Florida, where we stood with my mother and sister at my dying father's bedside. Following a brief visit and update on Dad's condition, I persuaded everyone to get some rest, relating that I would stay with Dad.

In the early hours of that morning after a lengthy one-sided conversation (he was unable to respond), I noticed a book on the nightstand, which had an intriguing title, very appropriate and timely for the present situation: *Gentle Closings: How To Say Goodbye To Someone You Love.* I picked it up and read it from cover to cover before sunrise. Not only did Ted Menten's counsel help me in those moments of despair, but they continue to influence me in offering care to others in similar situations. The most memorable words are poetic in nature and reflect the very essence of what it means to administer pastoral care:

> *"I believe that there is a supreme being.*
> *I like the idea of prayer.*
> *I believe that love gives the best return on investment.*
> *I believe in second chances, and third chances, and fourth chances.*
> *I believe that listening is essential to loving.*
> *I believe in grief and sorrow and wailing and tears flowing like Niagara Falls. Tears mean something. They mean we're alive and feeling.*
> *I believe that death is a friend, a fabulous dancer who will twirl me away in my last waltz.*
> *I believe in taking the time to say goodbye and not putting it off until another day.*
> *I believe in love, more than anything."*
>
> Ted Menten (1991, pp. 11–12)

Those words derived from lessons Menten learned from, primarily, dying children are meaningful for people of all ages. Something I find quite interesting, though, are many parallel thoughts to Menten contained in a prayer written by William G. Bartholome, a pediatrician, professor of medicine, and clinical ethicist, who also was taught many lessons from dying children, lessons which aided his own dying.

> *"The dying know best about living."*
>
> SLJ

Like Menten, the lectures and writings of Dr. Bartholome, especially this prayer, have greatly influenced my life's work. Therefore, as a way to honor Dr. Bartholome for instructing me in his dying and to provide the reader with insights for more effective pastoral care, I am reproducing, by permission, "A Prayer" (in Bartholome, 1999, pp. 27–28):

''The 'first last Christmas' in 1994 was so bittersweet. I felt in my bones that it would be my last. Yet it was Christmas, that most special time of year. There were many tears, but much joy. Little did I know that this was just the beginning of an incredible journey. A few weeks later, a force ... an incredible grace ... entered my life that would nourish and transform me in ways that I had never known. Although I barely knew it, our wedding was an awesome creation of life in the face of my illness. Pam tied her life together with mine in a way that has nourished me and grown me as a human beyond my wildest imaginings:

Thank you, God, for my partner, my wife, my Pam.

Over the course of these last four and a half years, I have become profoundly aware of the nature of my existence as a human being. I have come to realize that I exist suspended in, defined by, and nourished through a web of relationships. I know that I am because a man and woman conceived me into existence; because a woman bore me, birthed me, nourished me, cared for me, and protected me. From a wonderful mob of siblings I learned the lessons of sharing and loyalty and solidarity. From a long and troubled marriage and the searing pain of a divorce, I came to know that a needful love cannot maintain a relationship; that each of us is also called to sustain a solitary self.

From three incredible daughters and now a son, I have learned of the work, the joy, the pains, the satisfactions, the failings, and the letting go of being a father. From friends, from students, and from my patients and their families I have learned the meaning of living-in-relationship:

Thank you, God, for my parents, my siblings, my children, my web of being.

During this special time, I have been blessed in ways that I had never imagined possible. I have come to an awareness of myself and my life that few human beings are ever afforded the opportunity of developing. By making the choice to live in the light of death, I opened myself up to a process of discovery that continues to this very day. I am open to the beauty and intensity and richness and goodness of the world around me in ways that I had never experienced. I continue to be stunned and overwhelmed over and over again with this kind of living. I have come to know what it is like to actually live in the present ... to be totally alive in a moment of time:

Thank you, God, for this opportunity to be truly alive.

I have also been allowed to come to the discovery that this precious gift we call life is ours to make of what we will. This above ground 'fleshy phase' of our existence is a precious opportunity we are given to experience this world, to build bonds of caring and love with each other, to come to know what we are called to do here, and to create a legacy that will endure.

Over the last four years, I have attempted to share with all of you—but particularly with our children—my love, my spirit, my mind/heart. In the meditations I have shared with you, I have given you the gifts of my discoveries. I want more than anything to be for you a 'way-shower,' a guide, a teacher:

Thank you, God, for this opportunity to guide.

Living in this process has also grounded me in the awesome reality of Death. I have come to know the skeleton I am in the process of becoming in ways I never imagined possible. I feel His presence in my body in my every waking moment. Yet, I am no longer terrified by this reality. I have come to understand that it is Death that is the wellspring that drives our lives. Without Death, our lives would be pointless and empty. It is Death that wakes us to living. It is Death that prods us to discover and create ourselves and our lives in the few precious years we are given to share with each other here with our Mother Earth. I have encouraged you to embrace this strange traveling companion. His presence in your life will enrich your journey:

Thank you, God, for giving us this gift of life/death.

This journey has also opened up in me a renewed awareness of the relationship between my being and Father Sun and the Cosmos beyond. As I told you, living with Death on my shoulder has opened up in me an awareness of God's haunting presence. I know that God is. For me, beyond this awesome presence there is nothing but dense mystery. Yet, this one step of faith ... this simple conviction transforms me and my life.

At St. Andrew's Church, I now go to communion. I go to 'feed on Him in my heart through faith.' I am once again being spiritually nourished. Our service ends with the saints gathering around the altar and reciting an affirmation of purpose:

Thank you, God, for bringing me back to your presence.

I have been so blessed. You cannot possibly know the depth of my gratitude at having had these precious years to share with you. This special time of Christmas calls for celebration, joy, and acknowledgment of the multitude of gifts that fill our lives. This whole journey has been for me an incredible gift. I have had the opportunity to experience life and love and joy and peace beyond my wildest dreams:

Thank you, God, for this great gift.''

> *Dr. William G. Bartholome (1999, pp. 27–28)*

Additionally, I (SLJ) would be remiss not to mention the influence of Mitch Albom's *Tuesdays with Morrie* (1997) on my life. No doubt, you will have noticed quotes from his book throughout the pages of this book. Professor Morrie Schwartz made his own death *"the center of his days ... his final project"* in which he taught valuable lessons, not on how to die but how to live. Mitch Albom, Morrie's former student, came to his old professor's dying bedside on Tuesdays to get answers to a list of his own personal concerns: death, fear, aging, greed, marriage, family, society, forgiveness, a meaningful life (Albom, 1997, p. 66). The answer to all of those concerns can be summed up in these powerful words (Albom, 1997, pp. 92, 52, 91).

''Without love, we are birds with broken wings.''

''The most important thing in life is to learn how to give out love, and to let it come in.''

''Love each other or perish.''

> *Morrie Schwartz (Albom, 1997, pp. 92, 52, 91)*

I sincerely hope that Menten's, Bartholome's, and Albom's/Schwartz's words inspire and inform your caring presence as they have mine. However, you and, most especially, the people to whom you provide care may not share Menten's view of death as a "friend" or those of Bartholome's as the "wellspring that drives our lives" and a "strange traveling companion to embrace." On the contrary, for many, dying is the "valley of the shadow of death." Death itself is a thick fog that envelopes all that is familiar in the heart. Death is the enemy!

And so, in those anxious and stressful times for family and friends of the dying and/or the deceased, a pastoral care giver's presence is crucial.

"For in those moments, the one who comes stands beside those who find their dreams, hopes, and longings shattered by the awesome power of death and grief."

SLJ

This "one who comes" can offer the following things (Steven L. Jeffers, 2001, pp. 18–21):

- healing
- guiding
- sustaining
- reconciling.

It is the desire of the authors that as a result of reading and reflecting upon the contents of this book, you recognize these things:

- You can make a difference in the lives of the dying and the bereaved.
- You can empower the bereaved to give grief its voice.
- You can encourage the bereaved to go through grief.
- You can witness and applaud grievers' work by being their companion on the journey.

This last point is eloquently articulated by Harold Ivan Smith, in *Grieving the Death of a Friend* (1996):

"You want to know who helped me?
That's easy.
It wasn't the folks with the answers
or the folks with the pious clichés
and platitudes or
the folks with the advice.
No! It was those precious people
who listened all the way
to the end of my sentences
even when those babbled sentences
did not have periods.
It was those precious people
who let me sob and slobber
and moan and wail
and who simply sat with me
staring into the bottom of a coffee cup
as if the answers I needed

might be hiding there.
It was those who listened and nodded
and patted and hugged
and wept and waited with me
for this season called grief
to end.''

HIS (1996, pp. 107–108)

Finally, what is grief? It is a time to:

- remember
- reflect
- respect
- reconcile.

The ministry of presence can provide the opportunity for these things to happen.

''To Care Is to Be There!''

SLJ

Suggestions To Those Who Plan My Funeral

Use this form wisely. Consider well your entries. Be clear. Remember that you can neither explain nor change your comments after you are dead. However, do not feel compelled to complete this form in full. Keep in mind that you may harm your family by trying to give too much guidance. Help those you love to help themselves.

About My Family and Friends
These persons should be notified of my death as soon as possible:

Name/Relationship   Address   Phone #   email

_____
_____
_____

The following persons because of age, infirmity or other reasons should be notified personally by their clergy person, a friend, or an associate:

_____
_____

My ministers are —————————————————————————————
_____

Address, phone, email

My physicians are ————————————————————————————
_____

Address, phone, email

My attorney is ——————————————————————————————

Address, phone, email

My funeral director is ————————————————————————————

Address, phone, email

Material adapted from a document provided by former Kansas City Mayor and Methodist pastor, Emanuel Cleaver II.
Permission to reprint by author.

About Personal Data

This information will be needed for official certification. Accuracy is important. Claims, benefits, and legal procedures may be involved. This will become a permanent record and could be important to your family for many generations.

Full name: ————————————————————————————

Address: —————————————————————————————

City: ——————— County: ————————— State: ———————

Date of birth: ——————————— Birthplace: ———————

Occupation: ——————————— Business/Industry: —————

Employer: ———————————————————— Retired? ———

Union membership: ———————————————————
[Because of death benefits/funeral benefits]

Spouse: ————————————— Birthplace: ———————
　　　　　Full maiden name

Father: ————————————— Birthplace: ———————
　　　　　Full name

Stepfather: ——————————— Birthplace: ———————
　　　　　Full name

Mother: —————————— Birthplace: ———————
　　　　　Full maiden name

Stepmother: ——————— Birthplace: ———————
　　　　　Full maiden name

Social Security Number: ———————————————————

If ever employed by a railroad, list company and dates:

_____

If ever in Armed Services, Service Serial Number: ——————

Date of Service: ———————————————————————

If in Service under any other name: ——————————————

Attach a listing of biographical information: family relationships, faith congregation, fraternal, vocational, professional, club, or union affiliation, etc. Although not necessarily required, this might be useful.

Material adapted from a document provided by former Kansas City Mayor and Methodist pastor, Emanuel Cleaver II.
Permission to reprint by author.

About My Estate

I have ☐ I have not ☐ executed an estate planning document

If "yes" it is dated: ——————— and will be found: ———————

My executor is: ————————————————————————

My banks are: ————————————————————————

I have safety deposit box No. ——————— in ———————
                                                            Bank

It is held jointly with ————————————————————

Valuable papers not in this box will probably be found: ———————

(Attach separate notations, if advisable.)

About My Final Arrangements:

This form is intended to convey suggestions only. Except as hereinafter provided, your comments will be treated as suggestions only, not binding instructions. Unless otherwise indicated, your family will assume that this is only for their information, that you have not dictated firm decisions and that they are free either to confirm, or not confirm, your suggestions. It will be ONLY in connection with items that you ENCIRCLE AND INITIAL that it will be considered that your instructions shall prevail insofar as may be possible under the applicable laws.

Unless in conflict with the legal rights of others, I desire that the preferences of

————————————————————————
                            Name

my ——————— shall be given special consideration in connection with the ceremonial arrangements. If not possible, I designate ———————

————————————————————————
                            Name

my ——————— under the same conditions.

Material adapted from a document provided by former Kansas City Mayor and Methodist pastor, Emanuel Cleaver II.
Permission to reprint by author.

My preferred clergy persons: —————————————————————

_____

_____

_____

My preferred funeral directors: ————————————————————

_____

_____

_____

I prefer to have the ceremony held at —————————————————

_____

(faith congregation, funeral home, residence or other location)

I desire that final disposition be:

☐ Burial in ——————————————————————————————
                        Cemetery

Where I do ☐   do not ☐   have space.

If you do, describe: ——————————————————————————

Where is the cemetery lot certificate? ———————————————

☐ Entombment ————————— Where? ——————————————
☐ Cremation: Disposition of cremated remains: ————————————

_____

☐ Open casket

☐ Closed casket

I do ☐   do not ☐   desire to comment on the costs or qualities
of caskets, vaults, funeral services, etc.

If you do, make appropriate notations: ————————————————

_____

_____

Material adapted from a document provided by former Kansas City Mayor and Methodist pastor,
Emanuel Cleaver II.
Permission to reprint by author.

Outline as much detail of the funeral service as you feel necessary. Avoid such terms as "usual" or "customary." Such terms can be meaningless. You might want to suggest such things as scripture, music, or other ceremonial details.

_____
_____
_____
_____
_____

Note here the things which could enhance your rituals: (Clothing, hairdresser, glasses, bearers, flowers or anything else).

_____
_____
_____
_____

IF YOU DESIRE TO BE AN ORGAN/TISSUE DONOR AND/OR DONATE YOUR BODY FOR MEDICAL RESEARCH, YOU SHOULD DISCUSS THIS THOROUGHLY WITH YOUR FAMILY AND SUCH SHOULD BE DOCUMENTED IN AN ADVANCE DIRECTIVE.

I have ————— or have not ————— made payment of any costs. If yes, attach copy of receipt or a notation to where it will be found.

In subscribing to all the foregoing, I state that I have set forth these suggestions only in a spirit of helpfulness. I recognize that it is impossible for me to anticipate accurately all the circumstances that might affect my funeral. Therefore, excepting only such things as I may have encircled and initialed, the effect of which has already been noted in this folder, I specifically direct that the preferences of my family shall prevail.

Date: ————————————   ————————————————
                                    Signature

Witnesses

Name: ————————————   ————————————————
                                    Signature

Name: ————————————   ————————————————
                                    Signature

Notary

Name: ————————————   ————————————————
                                    Signature

Material adapted from a document provided by former Kansas City Mayor and Methodist pastor, Emanuel Cleaver II.

Permission to reprint by author.

Where To Find Help

Organizational Resources

American Academy of Bereavement
CMI Education Institute INC
892 Main Street
Buffalo, NY 14202
Phone: (800) 726-3888
www.cmieducation.org
www.bereavementacademy.org
The American Academy of Bereavement (AAB), a non-profit organization founded in 1993, is a national association devoted to the education, preparation and advancement of bereavement specialists. AAB serves as a stepping-stone for professional and personal growth in the field of bereavement. As an AAB member, you will have the opportunity to establish relationships with colleagues across the country. Through seminars, a yearly conference and networking, members are able to discuss the challenges and the gifts of this unique work.

Association for Death Education and Counseling
60 Revere Drive, Suite 500
Northbrook, IL 60062
Phone: (847) 509-0403
Fax: (860) 586-7550
www.adec.org
The Association for Death Education and Counseling provides death education, bereavement counseling, and support resources.

Centering Corporation
PO Box 4600
Omaha, NE 68104
Phone: (402) 553-1200
www.centeringcorp.com
The Centering Corporation is a non-profit organization dedicated to providing education and resources for the bereaved. Centering was founded in 1977 by Joy and Dr. Marvin Johnson.

Choice in Dying
200 Varick Street
New York, NY 10014-2507
Phone: (212) 366-5540 or (800) 989-9455
Fax: (212) 366-5337
Email: cid@choices.org
www.choices.org
Choice in Dying supplies information on laws affecting medical care and healthcare directives (living wills) in various states.

Hospice Association of America
228 Seventh Street, SE
Washington, DC 20003
Phone: (202) 546-4759
Fax: (202) 547-3540
Email: kpw@nahc.org
www.hospice-america.org
The Hospice Association of America seeks to heighten public awareness of hospice services as a viable component of the healthcare system.

Hospice Foundation of America
2001 South Street NW, Suite 300
Washington, DC 20009
Phone: (202) 638-5419
Fax: (202) 638-5312
www.hospicefoundation.org
The Hospice Foundation of America conducts programs to educate the public and healthcare workers on hospice-related issues. It also publishes free informational booklets.

National Alliance for Caregiving
4720 Montgomery Lane, Suite 642
Bethesda, MD 20814
Phone: (301) 718-8444
www.caregiving.org
The National Alliance for Caregiving is a nonprofit coalition of 25 national groups, which focus attention on family caregivers' issues. The Alliance conducts research, develops national programs and works to increase public awareness of the needs of family caregivers.

National Family Caregivers Association
10400 Connecticut Avenue, Suite 500
Kensington, MD 20895-2504
Phone: (301) 942-6230 or (800) 896-3650
Fax: (301) 942-2302
Email: info@nfcacares.org
www.nfcacares.org
The National Family Caregivers Association has several programs geared toward helping and informing caregivers: a newsletter entitled TAKE CARE; Caregiver-to-Caregiver Peer Support Network; Cards for Caregivers; Speaker's Bureau.

National Hospice and Palliative Care Organization
1700 Diagonal Road, Suite 300
Alexandria, VA 22314
Phone: (703) 243-5900 or (800) 658-8898
Email: drnho@cals.com
www.nhpco.org
The National Hospice and Palliative Care Organization provides referrals to local hospice services either directly or from its web site.

Rainbows
2100 Gold Road, Suite 370
Rolling Meadows, IL 60008-4231
Phone: (847) 952-1770 or (800) 266-3206
Fax: (847) 952-1774
www.rainbows.org
Rainbows runs support groups for people grieving the death of a loved one.
Informational guides and training for establishing peer support groups are also
available.

Suicide Awareness Voices of Education (SAVE)
7317 Cahill Road, Suite 207
Minneapolis, MN 55439-0507
Phone: (952) 946-7998 or (888) 511-7283
Email: save@winternet.com
www.save.org
SAVE's mission is to educate the public about suicide prevention and to speak for
suicide survivors. SAVE has educational programs on depression and suicide prevention, a school-based program for staff, students, and parents on suicide prevention, a
speakers' bureau, a quarterly brochure, as well as a number of publications and
public education tools.

National Suicide Hotline for Emergencies: (800) 784-2433

Online Resources

Death and Dying
www.death-dying.com
The Death and Dying web site provides phone numbers for support hotlines, grief
chat rooms, articles, and newsletters for people dealing with issues of bereavement.

Grief, Grief Recovery Golden Angels
www.groww.com
Grief, Grief Recovery Golden Angels supports the bereaved through a network of
chat rooms, message boards, and informational resources.

GriefNet
www.griefnet.org
GriefNet provides online support groups, bookstore information, and publishes
newsletters.

Willowgreen
www.willowgreen.com
Willowgreen is a leading provider of resources about illness, dying, loss and grief.
The company also produces numerous audiovisual materials.

The Robert Wood Johnson Foundation
www.rwj.org
The Robert Wood Johnson Foundation web site has a library of annual reports and
articles with the latest information about end-of-life issues.

Sources Cited

Aaron, W. F. (1999, December). "Funeral Service in the Year 2000." *The Director*, p. 5.

Aaron, W. F. (2000, January). "My New Year's Challenge." *The Director*, p. 4.

Albom, M. (1997). *Tuesdays with Morrie*. New York: Doubleday.

Alexander, V. (1991). *Words I Never Thought To Speak: Stories of Life in the Wake of Suicide*. New York: Lexington Books.

American Academy of Child and Adolescent Psychiatry. Facts for Families Section. *Teen suicide*. No. 10; updated July 2004. www.aacap.org

Anderson, R. C. (1985). *The Effective Pastor*. Chicago: Moody Press.

Ashe, A. and McCabe, A. (1995). *Arthur Ashe on Tennis: Strokes, Strategies, Traditions, Psychology, and Wisdom*. New York: Knopf.

Bagby, D. G. (1999). *Seeing Through Our Tears: Why We Cry, How We Heal*. Minneapolis: Augsburg.

Baha'is (1994). Publication of the Office of Public Information of the Baha'i International Community. Leicestershire, United Kingdom: Baha'i Publishing Trust of the United Kingdom.

Baker, J. E., Sedney, M. A., and Gross, E. (1992). "Psychological Tasks for Bereaved Children." *American Journal of Orthopsychiatry*, **62**(1): 105–116.

Balk, D. E. (1991) Death and Adolescent Bereavement: Current Research and Future Directions. Journal of Adolescent Research, **6**(1), pp. 7–27.

Balk, D. E. (2000). "Adolescents, Grief, and Loss." In K. J. Doka (ed.), *Living With Grief: Children, Adolescents, and Loss*, pp. 35–50. Philadelphia: Brunner/Mazel.

Bankoff, J. (1994, November 13). "A Tribute: A Man Who Sold You on Yourself." *The Atlanta Constitution*, p. D9.

Barrett, R.K. (1998) Sociocultural considerations for working with blacks, experiencing loss and grief. In: Doka, K. and Davidson, J.D. (eds) *Living With Grief: Who We Are, How We Grieve*, pp. 83–96. Philadelphia: Brunner/Mazel.

Bartholome, W. G. (1999). *Meditations* contained in *Bioethic Forum*, **16**(1). Kansas City: Midwest Bioethics Center.

Beattie, M. L. (1997). *Stop Being Mean to Yourself: A Story About Finding the True Meaning of Self-Love*. San Francisco: Harper.

Bereavement Services (1998). *It Means So Much To Know That Someone Cares*. La Cross, WI: Lutheran Hospital-La Crosse.

Bern-Klug, M. (1996). *Funeral Related Options and Costs: A Guide for Families*. Kansas City, KS: Center on Aging/FIP, University of Kansas Medical Center.

Bern-Klug, M., Ekerdt, D. J., and Wilkinson, D.S. (1999). "What Families Should Know About Funeral-related Costs: Implications for Social Work Practice." *Health & Social Work*, **24**(2), pp.128–137.

Bialosky, J. and Schulman, H. (1998, May 18). Review of *Wanting a Child: Twenty-Two Writers on Their Difficult But Mostly Successful Quest for Parenthood in a High-tech Age*. Time, pp. 76–79.

Blair, R. (1998). *The Funeral and Wedding Handbook*. Joplin, MO: College Press Publishing Company.

Bowlby, J. (1980). *Attachment and Loss: Loss, Sadness and Depression*. New York: Basic Books.

Brener, A. (1993). *Mourning and Mitzvah: A Guided Journal for Walking the Mourner's Path Through Grief to Healing*. Woodstock, VT: Jewish Lights.

Brody, J.E. (2004) Often, time beats therapy for treating grief. *New York Times* (electronic). http://www.nytimes.com/2004/01/27/health/Psychology/27BROD.html?el=5007&en=64837. Accessed 2 February 2007.

Brown, P. S. and Sefansky, S. (1995, October). "Enhancing Bereavement Care in the Pediatric ICU." *Critical Care Nurse*, **15**(5), pp. 59–64.

Burke, M. (1994). "Homosexuality as Deviance: The Case of a Gay Police Officer." *British Journal of Criminology*, **34**(2), pp. 192–203.

Burke, S. S. and Matsumoto, A. R. (1999). "Pastoral Care for Prenatal and Neonatal Health Care Providers." *Journal of Obstetric, Gynecologic, and Neonatal Nursing*, **22**, pp. 127–141.

Byock I. (2004) *The Four Things that Matter Most: A Book about Living*. New York: Free Press.

Capps, D. (2003). *Biblical Approaches to Pastoral Counselling*. Eugene, OR: Wipf & Stock Publishers.

Carroll, D. (1996, February 24). "Giving Parents a Chance To Heal." *The Kansas City Star*, pp. A1–A2.

Cassell, E. J. (1978). "Dying in a Technological Society. In R. Fulton, E. Markusen, G. Owen, and J. L. Scheiber (eds), *Death and Dying: Challenge and Change*. Reading: Addison-Wesley.

Centers for Disease Control and Prevention (1998, January 29). *Suicide in the United States*, pp. 1–3. Washington, DC: US Government Printing Office.

Clinebell, H. (1966/1984). *Basic Types of Pastoral Care and Counseling: Resources for the Ministry of Healing and Growth* (Rev. ed.). Nashville TN: Abingdon.

Coffin, H. S. Jr. (2006). Alex's Death. In: Bush, M. D. (ed.) *This Incomplete One: Words Occasioned by the Death of a Young Person*, pp. 53-60. Grand Rapids, MI: Eedermans.

Cook, A. S. and Oltjenbruns, K. A. (1998). *Dying and Grieving: Life-Span and Family Perspectives* (2nd edition.). Fort Worth: Harcourt Brace College Publishers.

Coolican, M. B., Stark, J., Doka, K. J., and Corr, C. A. (1994). "Education About Death, Dying, and Bereavement in Nursing Programs." *Nurse Educator*, **19**(6), pp. 35–40.

Corr, C. A. (1979). "Reconstructing the Face of Death." In H. Wass (ed.), *Dying: Facing the Facts*. New York: Hemisphere.

Corr, C. A. (1993). "Coping With Dying: Lessons That We Should and Should Not Learn From the Work of Elisabeth Kubler-Ross." *Death Studies*, **17**, pp. 69–83.

Corr, C. A. (2000). "What Do We Know About Grieving Children and Adolescents?" In K. J. Doka (ed.), *Living With Grief: Children, Adolescents, and Loss*, pp. 21–32. Philadelphia: Brunner/Mazel.

Corr, C. A., Nabe, C. M., and Corr, D. M. (1997). *Death and Dying Life and Living* (2nd edition). Pacific Grove, CA: Brooks/Cole Publishing.

Corr, C. A., Doka, K. J. and Kastenbaum, R. (1999). Dying and its interpreters: A review of selected literature and some comments on the state of the field. *Omega*. **39**(4): 239–259.

Creedy, A. (2000, May). "Year 2000 State of the Industry Analysis." *The American Funeral Director*, **112**(5), pp. 28–46.

Cuisinier, M., de Kleine, M., Kollee, L., Bethlehem, G., and de Grauuw, C. (1996). "Grief Following the Loss of a Newborn Twin Compared to a Singleton." *ACTA Pediatrics*, **85**, pp. 339–343.

DelBene, R., with Montgomery, M. and Montgomery, H. (1988). *A Time To Mourn: Recovering From the Death of a Loved One*. Nashville: The Upper Room.

DelBene, R. with Montgomery, M. and Montgomery, H. (1991). *From the Heart: Stories of a Pastor's Walk With His People*. Nashville: The Upper Room.

Digiulio, R. (1989). *Beyond Widowhood: From Bereavement to Emergence and Hope*. New York: Free Press.

Dobbins, R. D. (2000, Summer). "Widowed Too Young." *Enrichment*, **5**(3), pp. 70–72.

Doka, K. J. (1998). Disenfranchised grief. In: Doka, K. (ed.) *Disenfranchised Grief: Recognizing Hidden Sorrow*, pp. 3–11. Lexington, MA: Lexington Books.

Doka, K. J. (2000). "Using Ritual With Children and Adolescents." In K. J. Doka (ed.), *Living With Grief: Children, Adolescents, and Loss*, pp. 153–160. Philadelphia: Brunner/Mazel.

Doka, K. J. (2002). *Disenfranchised Grief: New Directions, Challenges and Strategies for Practice.* Champaign, IL: Research Press.

Dorland's Illustrated Medical Dictionary (1994). (Edition 28.) Philadelphia: W. B. Saunders.

Dowd, S. B., Poole, V. L., Davidhizar, R., and Giger, J. N. (1998). "Death, Dying and Grief in a Transcultural Context: Application of the Ginger and Davidhizar Assessment Model." *The Hospice Journal*, 13(4), pp. 33–56.

Downe-Wambolt, B. and Tamyln, D. (1997). "An International Survey of Death Education Trends in Faculties of Nursing and Medicine." *Death Studies*, **21**, pp. 177–188.

Edelman H. (1994) *Motherless Daughters: The Legacy of Loss.* New York: Addison-Wesley.

Everly, G. S. and Mitchell, J. T. (1999). *Critical Incident Stress Management* (2nd edition). Ellicott City, MD: Chevron Publishing Corporation.

Ewalt, P. L. and Perkins, L. (1979). "The Real Experience of Death Among Adolescents: An Empirical Study." *Social Casework*, **60**, pp. 547–551.

Farrell, P. (1997, August). "Ending the Stigma of Suicide." *The Director*, pp. 33–35.

Feifel, H. (1990). "Psychology and Death: Meaningful Rediscovery." *American Psychologist*, **45**(4): 537–543.

Feigenberg, L. (1980). *Terminal Care: Friendship Contracts With Dying Cancer Patients.* P. Hort (translator). New York: Brunner/Mazel.

Fitzgerald, H. (1994). *The Mourning Handbook.* New York: Simon and Schuster.

Flynn, T. (1987). "Dying as Doing: Philosophical Thoughts on Death and Authenticity." In M. A. Morgan and J. D. Morgan (eds), *Thanatology: A Liberal Arts Approach.* London, Ont: King's College.

Fulton R. and Fulton J. (1971). A psychosocial aspect of terminal care: Anticipatory grief. *Omega.* 2, pp. 91–99.

Gilbert R. B. (1998, February). "Take Off Your Shoes ... This Is Sacred Ground." *The Director*, pp. 10–14.

Goldman, L. (2000, May/June). "Suicide: How Can We Talk to the Children?" *The Forum*, pp. 6–9.

Goldstein, A. (1999, December 27). "Normal, Dull Days? No!" *Time*, p. 131.

Goodman, E. (1998). "Mourning Gets the Bum's Rush." *The Kansas City Star*, p. B7.

Goodwin, F. K. and Brown, G. L. (1989). "Risk Factors for Youth Suicide." In Alcohol, Drug Abuse, and Mental Health Administration, *Report on the Secretary's Task Force on Suicide*, Volume 1. Washington, DC: U.S. Department of Health and Human Services, Public Health Service, Alcohol Drug Abuse, and Mental Health Administration.

Hawkins, K. (2000, September 21). "Bereavement and the Native American." (Unpublished article.)

Hawley L. III (1990). "Grief and the funeral director: We, too, hurt sometimes." In: Pine V.R., Margolis O.S., Doka, K, Kutscher A.H., Schaefer, D.J., Siegel, M-E and Cherico, D.J. (eds.) *Unrecognized and Unsanctioned Grief: The Nature and Counseling of Unacknowledged Loss.*, pp. 158-160. Springfield, IL: Charles C. Thomas.

Husain, S. A. (1990). "Current Perspective on the Role of Psychological Factors in Adolescent Suicide." *Psychiatric Annals*, **20**, pp. 122–127.

International Commission on English in the Liturgy (1990). Rev. study ed. Chicago: Liturgy Training Publications.

Jamison, K. R. (1999). *Night Falls Fast: Understanding Suicide.* New York: Vintage.

Jeffers, S. L. (2001). *Finding a Sacred Oasis in Illness: Pastoral Care Package*, Volume I. Overland Park, KS: Leathers Publishing.

Jennings, K. (1998, September 29). "My Perspective: Be a Man." *The Advocate*, p. 11.

Johnson, C. J. and McGee, M. G. (1998). *How Different Religions View Death and Afterlife*. Philadelphia: The Charles Press.

Johnson, E. A. (1999). *Friends of God and Prophets: A Feminist Theological Reading of the Communion of Saints*. New York: Continuum.

Johnson J. (2006). Personal correspondence to Harold Ivan Smith. 25 October.

Jordan, J. R. (2000, May/June). "Is Suicide Bereavement Different?" *The Forum*, pp. 2–3.

Kastenbaum, R. J. (1969). "Death and Bereavement in Later Life." In A. H. Kutscher (ed.), *Death and Bereavement*. Springfield, IL: Charles C. Thomas.

Kastenbaum,. R. J. (1986). Death, Society and Human Experience (3e). Columbus, OH: Charles Merrill; cited in Corr, C. A. (1993) Coping with Dying: Lessons that we should and should not learn from the work of Elisabeth Kublier-Ross. *Death Studies*. **17**, p.70.

Kastenbaum, R. J. (1998). *Death, Society and Human Experience* (6e). Boston: Allyn & Bacon.

Kastenbaum, R. J. (2000). "The Kingdom Where Nobody Dies." In: Doka, K. J. (ed.) *Living With Grief: Children, Adolescents and Loss*, pp. 5-20. Philadelphia: Brunner/Mazel.

Kastenbaum, R. and Aisenberg, R. (1972). *The Psychology of Death*. New York: Springer.

Kellner, K. and Lake, M. (1990). "Grief Counseling." In R. Knuppel and J. Drukker (eds), *High Risk Pregnancy: A Team Approach*, pp. 717–731. Philadelphia: W. B. Saunders.

Kennell, J. H., Slyter, H., and Klaus, M. H. (1970). "The Mourning Response of Parents to the Death of a Newborn Infant." *New England Journal of Medicine*, **283**, pp. 344–349.

Kimble, D. L. (1991). "Neonatal Death: A Descriptive Study of Fathers' Experience." *Neonatal Network*, **9**(8), pp. 45–50.

Kippel, R. (2000, May/June). "Suicide in Law Enforcement: It's Personal." *The Forum*, pp. 11–12.

Kooten, H., with Flowers, C. (2000). *Golden Men: The Power of Gay Midlife*. New York: Avon.

Kramer, J. (1970). *Lombardi: Winning is the Only Thing*. New York: World.

Kreindler, J. D., Rabbi (2000). "Jewish Tradition and Laws Concerning Death and Mourning." (Unpublished paper.)

Krietemeyer, B. and Heiney, S. P. (1992). "Storytelling as a Therapeutic Technique in Group for School Age Oncology Patients." *Children's Health Care*, **21**, pp. 14–20.

Krug, E. (1997, February 7). Cited in "Murder, Suicide Taking More of U. S. Youths." *The Kansas City Star*, p. A-9.

Kubler-Ross, E. (1969). *On Death and Dying*. New York: MacMillan.

L'Engle, M. (1998). *Two Part Invention: The Story of a Marriage*. New York: Farrar, Straus & Giroux.

Lewis, C. S. (1961). *A Grief Observed*. New York: Bantam.

Limbo, R. K. and Wheeler, S. R. with Hessel, S. T. (1986). *When a Baby Dies: A Handbook for Healing and Helping*. La Crosse, WI: Lutheran Hospital.

Lindemann, E. (1986). *Beyond Grief: Studies in Crisis Intervention*, pp. 59–78. New York: Jason Aronson.

Lipson, J. G., Dibble, S. L. and Minarik, P. A. (eds.) (1996). *Culture and Nursing Care: A Pocket Guide*. San Francisco, CA: University of California San Francisco Nursing Press.

Logan, K (bd) *Creating a Ritual*. Kansas City, MO: Kansas City Hospice document.

Long, T. G. (1997, October). "The American Funeral Today—Trends and Issues." *The Director*, pp. 10–16.

Long, T. G. (1999). "Why Jessica Mitford Was Wrong." *Theology Today*, **55**(4), pp. 496–509.

Lothrop, H. (1997). *Help, Comfort and Hope After Losing your Baby in Pregnancy or the First Year*. Tucson, AZ: Fisher Books.

Lynch, T. (1997). *The Undertaking: Life Studies From the Dismal Trade*. New York: Norton.

Madigan, T. (2006). *I'm Proud of You; My Friendship with Fred Rogers*. New York: Gothan Books.

Mahan, M. (1999, July/August). "Bereaved Children and Secondary Losses." *The Forum*, **24**(4), p. 5.

Malikow, M. (1999, April). "Suicide Postvention." *The Director*, pp. 40, 42, 44.

Manning, D. (1979). *Don't Take My Grief Away*. San Francisco: Harper and Row.

Martin, T and Doka, K. J. (1996). Masculine Grief. In: Doka, K. J. (ed.) *Living with Grief After Sudden Loss: Suicide, Homicide, Accident, Heart Attack, Stroke*. Washington DC: Taylor & Francis.

Martin, T. L. and Doka, K. J. (1998). Revisiting masculine grief. In: Doka, K. J. and Davidson, J. D. (eds.) *Living With Grief: Who We Are, How We Grieve*, pp.132–42. Philadelphia: Brunner/Mazel.

Martin, T. L. and Doka, K. J. (2000). *Men Don't Cry ... Women Do: Transcending Stereotypes of Grief*. Philadelphia: Brunner/Mazel.

Marzuk, P. M. (1994). "Suicide and Terminal Illness." *Death Studies*, **18**, pp. 497–505.

Mathewes-Green, F. (1999). *At the Corner of East and Now*. New York: Jeremy T. Tarcher.

McCullough, D. (1992). *Truman*. New York: Simon & Schuster.

McKormick M. (2000). That Personal Touch. *The American Funeral Director*. **20**, p. 23.

McMahon, M. P. (2000, May/June). "What Can You Do? The Journey Continues." *The Forum*, p. 10.

Meigs J. T. (1984) *Home Life*. Nashville, TN: The Southern Baptist Convention.

Menke, J. and McClead, R. (1990). "Perinatal Grief and Mourning." *Advances in Pediatrics*, **37**, pp. 261–283.

Menten, T. (1991). *Gentle Closings: How To Say Goodbye To Someone You Love*. Philadelphia: Running Press.

Miles, A. (1995, May/June). "Dealing With the Death of a Child." *The American Journal of Hospice & Palliative Care*, **2**, pp. 36–40.

Miller, J. (1996). *How Will I Get Through the Holidays: 12 Ideas for Those Whose Loved One Has Died*. Fort Wayne, IN: Willowgreen Publishing.

Minarik, P. A., Dribble S., Lipson, J. (1996) *Culture and Nursing Care: A Pocket Guide*. San Francisco: University of California San Francisco School of Nursing.

Minutaglio, B. (1999). *First Son: George W. Bush and the Bush Family Dynasty*. New York: Time Books/Random House.

Mir, A. R. MD (2001, February). "An Islamic Perspective on Dealing with Death." (Unpublished paper.)

Mitchell, J. T. (1999). "We Remember!" *Life Net*. **10**(4). A publication of the International Critical Incident Stress Foundation Inc., p. 5.

Mitchell, J. T. and Everly, G. S. (1997). *Critical Incident Stress Debriefing: An Operations Manual* (2nd edition revised). Ellicott City, MD: Chevron Publishing Corporation.

Mufson, L., Moreau, D., Weissman, M. M., and Klerman, G. L. (1993). *Interpersonal Psychotherapy for Depressed Adolescents*. New York: Guilford.

Murphy, N. M. (1999). *The Wisdom of Dying: Practices for Living*. Boston: Element.

National Institute of Mental Health (2005). In Harms Way: Suicide in America. http://www.nimh.nih.gov/public/harmaway.cfm?Output=Print. Accessed 23 July 2005.

Neeld, E. H. (1990). *Seven Choices: Taking the Steps to New Life After Losing Someone You Love*. New York: Delta Books.

Neimeyer, R. A. (1998). *Lessons of Loss: A Guide to Coping*. New York: McGraw-Hill/Premis Custom Publishing.

Nelson B. (2001, April 4). "Buddhism, Death and Dying." A presentation given at Johnson County Community College as part of a Symposium for healthcare professionals entitled *Religious Diversity in Health Care: A Foundation for a Holistic Care*.

NFO Research (1999). "When a Child Dies: A Survey of Bereaved Parents." *Forum*, **25**(6), pp. 1, 10–11.

Nighswonger, C. (1972, June). "Ministry to the Dying as a Learning Encounter." *The Journal of Pastoral Care*, **26**.

Nikhilananda, Swami (translator) (1944). *The Bhagavad Gita*. New York: Ramakrishna-Vivekananda.

Nuland, S. B. (1994). *How We Die: Reflections on Life's Final Chapter*. New York: Knopf.

Nuland, S. B. (2003). *Lost in America: My Journey with my Father*. New York: Alfred N. Knopf.

Oates W. (1972). *Anxiety in Christian Experience*. Waco, TX: Word.

Oden, T. (1983). *Pastoral Theology: Essentials of Ministry*. San Francisco: Harper & Row.

O'Neill, B. (1998). "A Father's Grief: Dealing With Stillbirth." *Nursing Forum*, **33**(4), pp. 33–37.

Outlaw, E. (2000). "Creative Ministry." (Unpublished article.)

Page-Lieberman, J. and Hughes, C. B. (1990). "How Fathers Perceive Perinatal Death." MCN: *American Journal of Maternal/Child Nursing*, **15**, pp. 320–323.

Parachin, V. M. (1998a, February). "Grief Relief: How Our Friends Helped After a Death to Suicide." *The Director*, pp. 4, 6, 8.

Parachin, V. M. (1998b, May). Grief Relief: How to Help a Grieving Teenager. *The Director*, pp. 14, 16.

Parachin, V. M. (1998c, July). "The Mourning After: Ten Healing Steps for Grieving Men." *The Director*, pp. 20, 22, 24.

Parachin, V.M. (2006, July). "Children and Loss: Eight Ways That You, or the Families You Serve, Can Help Children Cope With the Reality of Death." *The Director*, pp. 60–65.

Parkes, C. M. (1972). *Bereavement: Studies of Grief in Adult Life*. New York: International Universities Press.

Parsons, T., Fox, R. C., and Lidz, V.M. (1973). "The 'Gift of Life' and its Reciprocation." In A. Mack (ed.), *Death in American Experience*. New York: Schocken.

Pattison, E. M. (1977). *The Experience of Dying*. Englewood Cliffs, NJ: Prentice Hall.

Perret, G. (1999). *Eisenhower*. New York: Random House.

Pinchon, F. (1968). *Life After Death*. Wilmette, IL: Baha'i Publishing Trust.

Rando, T. A. (1984). *Grief, Dying and Death: Clinical Interventions for Care Givers*. Champaign, IL: Research Press.

Rando, T. A. (1986). *Parental Loss of a Child*. Champaign, IL: Research Press.

Rando, T. A. (1992–93). "The Increasing Prevalence of Complicated Mourning: The Onslaught is Just Beginning." *Omega*, **26**(1), pp. 43–59.

Rando, T. A. (1993). *Treatment of Complicated Mourning*. Champaign, IL: Research Press.

Rando, T. A. (ed.) (2000). *Clinical Dimensions of Anticipatory Mourning: Theory and Practice in Working with the Dying, Their Loved Ones and Their Caregivers*. Champaign, IL: Research Press.

Rando, T.A. (2002). *Clinical Dimensions of Anticipatory Mourning*. Presentation. Overland Park, KS: Kansas City Hospice.

Raphael, B. (1983). *The Anatomy of Bereavement*. New York: Basic Books.

"Redeeming Funerals." (1999, April 26). *Christianity Today*, p. 27.

Rich, T. R. (1996). "Judaism 101: Life, Death and Mourning." www.jewfaq.org/death.htm

Rinpoche, S. (1993). *The Tibetan Book of Living and Dying*. San Francisco: Harper.

Rosen, H. (1984–85). "Prohibitions Against Mourning in Childhood Sibling Loss." *Omega*, **15**, pp. 307–316.

Saint Francis Xavier Church. (1996). *A Guide to Funeral Planning at Saint Francis Xavier Church.* Kansas City, MO.

Scheinerman, A. R. (2000). "The Jewish Life Cycle: Death." Use: http://ezra.mts.jhu.edu/~rabbiars/life-cycle/death.html. Click on Rabbi Scheinerman's Judaism website, then click on "mourning" from menu.

Schlosser, E. (1997, September). "A Grief Like No Other." *The Atlantic Monthly*, pp. 37+.

Schubiner, H. (1991, June). "How To Identify a Suicidal Teen." *Medical Aspects of Human Sexuality*, pp. 51–52.

Shneidman, E. S. (1980/1995). *Voices of Death.* New York: Harper & Row/Kodansha International.

Sims, D. (1991). "A Model For Grief-Intervention and Death Education in Public Schools." In J. D. Morgan (ed.), *Youth, People and Death*, pp. 185–190. Philadelphia: The Charles Press.

Sittser, G. L. (1995). *A Grace Disguised: How the Soul Grows Through Loss.* Grand Rapids: Zondervan Publishing House.

Smith, H. I. (1996). *Grieving the Death of a Friend.* Minneapolis: Augsburg.

Smith Harold Ivan (2001) *ABCs of Health Bereavement: Light for a Dark Journey*, p. 56. Shawnee Mission, KS: Shawnee Mission Medical Center.

Smith, K. (1999, November). "Ten Tips for Tough Times." *The Director*, p. 32.

Speece, M. W. and Brent, S. B. (1996). "The Development of Children's Understanding of Death." In C. A. Corr and D. M. Corr (eds), *Handbook of Childhood Death and Bereavement*, pp. 29–50. New York: Springer.

Stanford, C. (1999). "Guidelines for A Buddhist Funeral." (Unpublished article.)

Staudacher, C. (1991). *Men and Grief: A Guide for Men Surviving the Death of a Loved One.* Oakland, CA: New Harbinger Publications.

Steere, D. A. (2002). *The Supervision of Pastoral Care.* Eugene, OR: Wipf & Stock Publishers.

Stimming, M. T. (2000, March 8). "Grace in the Face of Suicide." *Christian Century*, pp. 272–274.

Stroebe, M. (1992–93). "Coping With Bereavement: A Review of the Grief Work Hypothesis." *Omega*, **26**(1), pp. 19–42.

Strommen, M. P. and A. I. (1993). *Five Cries of Grief: One Family's Journey to Healing After the Tragic Death of a Son.* New York: HarperCollins.

Switzer, D. K. (1974). *The Minister as Crisis Counselor.* Nashville: Abingdon.

Tillich, P. (1959, October). "The Theology of Pastoral Care." *Pastoral Psychology*, Vol. 10, Nov. 97, pp. 21–26.

Toray, T. (2000, May/June). "Death by Any Other Name." *The Forum*, pp. 4–5.

U.S. Census Bureau (1999). *Statistical Abstract of the United States: 1999.* Washington, DC: U.S. Government Printing Office.

U.S. Census Bureau (2006). *Statistical Abstract of the United States: 2006*, p. 79. Washington, DC: U.S. Government Printing Office.

Vogel, G. E. (1996). *A Caregiver's Handbook to Perinatal Loss.* St. Paul: A Place to Remember.

Voide, E. (1998, February). "Children Should Be Seen and Heard." *The Director*, pp. 24, 26, 28.

Walfoort, N. (1998). Newcomers Fuel Increase in Housing Services. *The Louisville Courier Journal*, pp. A1, A5.

Wallerstedt, C. and Higgins, P. (1996). "Facilitating Perinatal Grieving Between the Mother and the Father." *Journal of Obstetric, Gynecologic, and Neonatal Nursing*, **25**(5), pp. 389–394.

Webb, N. B. (2000). "Play Therapy to Help Bereaved Children." In K. J. Doka (ed.), *Living With Grief: Children, Adolescents, and Loss*, pp. 153–160. Philadelphia: Brunner/Mazel.

Weisman, A. D. (1972). *On Dying and Denying: A Psychiatric Study of Terminality.* New York: Behavioral Publications.

Wheat, R. (1996, February). "Shattered Dreams: Be Careful What You Say." *Home Life*, pp. 31–33.

White, J. F. (1980/1990). *Introduction to Christian Worship* (revised edition). Nashville: Abingdon.

Wilken, C. S. and Powell, J. (1993). *Learning to Live Through Loss: Understanding Men Who Grieve*. Manhattan, KS: Cooperative Extension Service, Kansas State University.

Wiltshire, S. F. (1994). *Seasons of Grief and Grace*. Nashville: Vanderbilt University Press.

Wolfelt, A. D. (1994). *Creating Meaningful Funeral Rituals: A Guide for Care Givers*. Fort Collins, CO: Compassion Press.

Wolfelt, A. D. (1996). *Healing the Bereaved Child: Grief Gardening, Growth Through Grief and Other Touchstones for Care Givers*. Fort Collins, CO: Compassion Press.

Wolfelt, A. D. (1997a). *The Journey Through Grief*. Fort Collins, CO: Compassion Press.

Wolfelt, A. D. (1997b). "Educating the Families You Serve with a Service Room." *The Director*. 30, 32, 34.

Woodward, K. L. with Underwood, A. (1998, September 22). "The Ritual Solution." *Newsweek*, p. 62.

Worden, J. W. (1991). *Grief Counseling and Grief Therapy: A Handbook for the Mental Health Practitioner* (2nd edition). New York: Springer Publishing.

Worden, J. W. (1996). *Children and Grief: When a Parent Dies*. New York: Guilford.

Worden, J. W. (2001). *Grief Counseling and Grief Therapy: A Handbook for the Mental Health Practitioner* (3rd edition). New York: Springer Publishing.

Yancey, V. Midwest Bioethics Center's *Compassion Sabbath* Kickoff. September 1999. Material attributed to Dr Yancey taken from her keynote presentation.

Zedek, M. (1999, September 22). "The Uses of Ritual." Compassion Sabbath. Grace and Holy Trinity Cathedral, Kansas City, MO.

Recommended Reading

- Albom, Mitch (1997). *Tuesdays with Morrie*. New York: Doubleday.
  Rarely has a book on death been a bestseller for several years on *The New York Times* bestseller list. But there was never quite a person like Morrie Schwartz. Through the eyes of his student and friend, Mitch Albom, we learn a great deal about the last months of a dying man's life.

- Atkinson, Donald R. and Hackett, Gail (eds) (2004). *Counseling Diverse Populations* (3rd edition). Boston: McGraw-Hill.
  This significant book addresses the challenges of counseling non-ethnic minorities in four categories: people with disabilities, older adults, women, and sexual minorities. Particularly helpful for acquainting the pastoral care provider with language and issue sensitivity that can become barriers to effectiveness.

- Attig, Thomas (2000). *The Heart of Grief: Death and the Search for Lasting Love*. New York: Oxford University Press.
  This book offers profound insights into the meaning of death and how to maintain a lasting love with those who have died. The book helps us learn to love in their absence just as we loved in their presence.

- Bagby, Daniel G. (1999). *Seeing Through Our Tears: Why We Cry, How We Heal*. Minneapolis, MN: Augsburg.
  Death is only one of many losses we experience. But death can be tag-teamed with other losses. Bagby insists that we can find God through those losses.

- Baugher, Bob and Jordan, Jack (2002). *After Suicide Loss: Coping With Your Grief*. Newcastle, WA: Robert Baugher.
  This griever-friendly book is readable and suitable for the family member or friend who is experiencing grief following a suicide.

- Bernardin, Joseph, Cardinal (1997). *The Gift of Peace*. Chicago, IL: Loyola Press.
  In the final two months of his life, Cardinal Bernadin of Chicago shares his experience of "losing" the battle with cancer. He also relates about the "gift" of a peaceful death.

- Byock, Ira (2004). *The Four Things That Matter Most: A Book About Living*. New York: Free Press.
  This book is a compendium of the lessons Byock learned from a quarter century working in hospice and palliative care.

- *Caring to Help Others: A Training Manual for Preparing Volunteers to Assist Caregivers of Older Adults* (2000).
  Eisai, Inc., Teaneck, New Jersey, a research-based global pharmaceutical company, sponsored the development of this training manual. It is a comprehensive, collaborative resource of incredible worth. The manual can be accessed on line at www.caringtohelpothers.com. A hard copy can be obtained from Caring to Help Others, PO Box 212, Ridgefield Park, New Jersey 07660.

- Carmack, Betty J. (2003). *Grieving the Death of a Pet.* Minneapolis: Augsburg Books.
  The relationship between individuals and pets is unique and so is the grief experience when a pet dies. Many are stunned by the intensity and duration of this loss. This book is an important resource for permissioning grief following a pet's death.

- Corr, Charles A., Nabe, Clyde M., and Corr, Donna M. (1997). *Death and Dying Life and Living* (2nd edition). Pacific Grove, CA: Brooks/Cole Publishing.
  This is an "A to Z" compendium on dying, death, and bereavement used in many universities. If you have a question about death, you will find at least part of the answer here.

- Davis, Laura (2002). *I Thought We'd Never Speak Again: The Road From Estrangement to Reconciliation.* New York: HarperCollins.
  Given the numbers of dysfunctional families, this "mapbook" will be of great use to pastoral care givers who must deal with families in their worse moments.

- Doka, Kenneth (1989). *Disenfranchised Grief: Recognizing Hidden Sorrow.* Lexington, MA: Lexington Books.
  In this book, the author discusses the unique situation of bereaved survivors whose loss is not, or cannot be, openly acknowledged, publicly mourned, or socially supported.

- Doka, Kenneth (ed.) (2002). *Disenfranchised Grief: New Directions, Challenges and Strategies.* Champaign, IL: Research Press.
  This volume offers the most current theoretical development and clinical practice in disenfranchised grief, a concept first presented by Doka in 1989. Sections include a theoretical overview, tools and techniques for clinical interventions, illustrations of practice, and implications for education and policy.

- Dunn, Hank (1999). *Light in the Shadows: Meditations While Living With a Life-Threatening Illness.* Herndon, VA: A & A Publishers, Inc.
  This little book is about finding hope in hopeless situations, living a meaningful life in the light of death, how to experience a connection to the eternal. This is a must read for any person ministering to those at the end of life.

- Dunn, Hank (2001). *Hard Choices for Loving People* (4th edition). Herndon, VA: A & A Publishers, Inc.
  This is an incredibly practical and useful booklet to help patients and families make decisions about life-prolonging procedures. The concluding chapter addresses the emotional and spiritual struggles with end-of-life decisions.

- Evans, Richard Paul (1999). *The Dance.* New York: Simon & Schuster.
  Dancing marks the rites of passage through a daughter's life. Her father is always watching her performances. But after his death, will she be able to dance again?

- Fitzgerald, Helen (1994). *The Mourning Handbook.* New York: Simon & Schuster.
  A death results in feelings, anxieties and concerns that lead to our "How do I/ how will I ...?" questions. Fitzgerald offers readers practical advice on what to expect and how to cope. This book is a guidebook for the journey through grief.

- Fitzgerald, Helen (2000). *Grief at Work: A Manual of Policies and Practices.* Washington, DC: American Hospice Foundation.
  A death of a colleague in the workplace or a death in a coworker's family can be a challenging experience. Fitzgerald offers a comprehensive guide to being supportive.

- Fox, Mem (1994). *Wilfred Gordon McDonald Partridge.* New York: Harcourt and Brace.
  Wilfred Gordon McDonald Partridge lives next door to an "old people's home." There he learns that memories are something that makes you laugh or something that makes you cry, or something as "precious as gold." This book will help children talk about their memories of a loved one.

- Gilbert, Richard (1999). *Finding Your Way After Your Parent Dies.* Notre Dame, IN: Ave Maria Press.
  This book offers wise guidance for those who have lost one or both parents.

- Gootman, Marilyn E. (1994). *When a Friend Dies: A Book for Teens About Grieving and Healing.* Minneapolis, MN: Free Spirit Publishing.
  Death can be very confusing to a teen, particularly when a friend dies. This book is a griever's friend—easily readable for adolescents.

- Guest, A. G. (Compiler) (1993). *A Little Book of Comfort: An Anthology of Grief and Love.* Grand Rapids, MI: Marshall Pickering/HarperCollins.
  Sooner or later grief's shadow touches all of us. This book is a compilation of "soul soothing" quotations that will be useful to the funeral/memorial service planner as well as the griever.

- Harris, Jill Werman (ed.) (1999). *Remembrances and Celebrations: A Book of Eulogies, Elegies, Letters, and Epitaphs.* New York: Pantheon Books.
  You have been asked to do a eulogy at a funeral. This book offers a wide range of samples of materials from the funeral services of the famous and not so famous.

- Jeffers, Steven L. (2001). *Finding a Sacred Oasis in Illness: Pastoral Care Package,* Volume I. Overland Park, KS: Leathers Publishing.
  There continues to be an increasing interest in the role spirituality plays in health. Data suggests that patients and families want their spiritual issues addressed because, for many, spiritual beliefs play a major role in how they cope with stress, suffering and grief. This book offers practical insights and situation-specific illustrations on how to effectively meet people's spiritual needs from multiple religious traditions during difficult times.

- Kauffman, Jeffrey (ed.) (2002). *Loss of the Assumptive World: A Theory of Traumatic Loss.* New York: Brunner-Routledge.
  A traumatic death can challenge, if not shatter, the assumptions by which an individual lives – children will bury parents. Thus, sometimes both the death and the assumption have to be grieved and addressed.

- Lewis, C. S. (1961). *A Grief Observed.* New York: Bantam.
  C. S. Lewis became something of an expert on grief during World War II. Then, after four years of marriage to Joy Davidson, her death made him a griever. In 80 pages, Lewis gives people permission to do their grief. This book has comforted millions of people. A must-read classic.

- Lynch, Thomas (1997). *The Undertaking: Life Studies From the Dismal Trade*. New York: Norton.
  Few people understand death like Thomas Lynch, a fourth-generation funeral director. His insights into death and stories about the thousands of people he has buried are an alternative to the "Digger O'Dell" mentality toward funeral directors.

- Magida, Arthur J. (ed.) (1996). *How To Be A Perfect Stranger: A Guide to Etiquette in Other People's Religious Ceremonies* (Vol. 1). Woodstock, VT: Jewish Lights Publishing.
  In today's multicultural society, sooner or later you will have a friend who does not practice your faith (or any faith). How can you enter, what the author calls, "unfamiliar territory" without offense? This practical handbook offers advice not only on funerals but also on weddings, births of new babies, and special ways of practicing various faith traditions' rituals. The book includes information on Buddhism, Hinduism, Islam, Judaism, as well as selected Christian denominations.

- Manning, Doug (1979). *Don't Take My Grief Away*. San Francisco: Harper and Row.
  The title says it all: "Don't let anyone take away, limit, diminish, or disenfranchise your grief."

- Martin, Terry and Doka, Kenneth (2001). *Men Don't Cry, Women Do: Transcending Gender Stereotypes on Grief*. Philadelphia: Brunner-Mazel.
  This book analyses myths about gender and grief. The book explains the strengths and limitations of grieving styles that are related to but not determined by gender. *Men Don't Cry, Women Do* includes a foreword by Dr. Therese A. Rando.

- Matlins, Stuart M. (ed.) (2000). *The Perfect Stranger's Guide to Funerals and Grieving Practices: A Guide to Etiquette in Other People's Religious Ceremonies*. Woodstock, VT: Skylight Paths Publishing.
  Grieving a colleague or friend's death can be awkward when one is unfamiliar with their religious or spiritual tradition. This helpful paperback gives a thumbnail sketch for being a compassionate, supportive presence.

- Matlins, S. M. and Magida, A. J. (eds) (1997). *How To Be A Perfect Stranger: A Guide to Etiquette in Other People's Religious Ceremonies* (Vol 2). Woodstock, VT: Jewish Lights Publishing.
  This second volume offers insights into religious practices of smaller Christian denominations. The reader gains insight into attending such events as weddings, funerals and committals.

- Matlins, S. M. and Magida, A. J. (eds) (2006). *How To Be A Perfect Stranger: The Essential Religious Etiquette Handbook* (4th edition). Woodstock, VT: Skylight Paths Publishing.
  This version is updated and revised with an expanded glossary of common religious terms and names and a new section focusing on the meaning of popular religious symbols. This easy-to-read guidebook helps the well-meaning guest to feel comfortable, participate to the fullest extent possible, and avoid violating anyone's religious principles—while enriching their own spiritual understanding. Faith traditions addressed in this edition include: African American Methodist

Churches ● Assemblies of God ● Bahá'í ● Baptist ● Buddhist ● Christian Church (Disciples of Christ) ● Christian Science (Church of Christ, Scientist) ● Churches of Christ ● Episcopalian and Anglican ● Hindu ● Islam ● Jehovah's Witnesses ● Jewish ● Lutheran ● Mennonite/Amish ● Methodist ● Mormon (Church of Jesus Christ of Latter-day Saints) ● Native American/First Nations ● Orthodox Churches ● Pentecostal Church of God ● Presbyterian ● Quaker (Religious Society of Friends) ● Reformed Church in America/Canada ● Roman Catholic ● Seventh-day Adventist ● Sikh ● Unitarian Universalist ● United Church of Canada ● United Church of Christ.

- McIntee, Jeanne Daly (1998). *To Comfort, To Honor: A Guide to Personalizing Rituals for the Passing of a Loved One.* Minneapolis, MN: Augsburg.
  In this book, the reader will learn how to personalize a service.

- Menten, Ted (1991). *Gentle Closings*: *How To Say Goodbye To Someone You Love.* Philadelphia: Running Press.
  This book is about people who have said good-bye, and how they did it. In these pages, you will see how people pushed aside their despair to rejoice in shared memories and face death with warmth, frankness, and even humor. These stories can provide anyone with ideas, reassurance, and the courage needed at such a critical time.

- Miller, James (1996). *How Will I Get Through the Holidays: 12 Ideas for Those Whose Loved One Has Died.* Fort Wayne, IN: Willowgreen Publishing.
  How can I celebrate with a broken heart? Miller offers a dozen simple ideas for the first holidays.

- Munsch, Robert (1986). *Love You Forever.* Willowdale, Ontario, Canada: Firefly Books.
  One of the classics in children's literature, beloved by adults as well as children, is about a mother who, in various stages of her life, promises, ''I will love you forever, I will love you for always.''

- Rupp, Joyce (1988). *Praying Our Goodbyes.* Notre Dame, IN: Ave Maria Press.
  ''Who can pray at a time like this?'' grievers often ask. Yet, the songs say, ''Take it to the Lord in prayer.'' The author argues that instead of running from our losses, we reflect on them, engage them, and pray them. The facts do not change, but we change through prayer.

- Rylant, Cynthia (1995/1997). *Dog Heaven and Cat Heaven.* New York: Blue Sky Press.
  Great illustrations and a creative story line create animal companions for pet lovers of any age who are grieving the death of a pet.

- Searle, Edward (1993). *In Memoriam: A Guide to Modern Funeral and Memorial Services.* Boston: Skinner House.
  If you are facing the loss of someone you know or having to plan a service (funeral or memorial), this comprehensive guide gives practical advice and ideas.

- Sittser, Gerald L. (1995). *A Grace Disguised: How the Soul Grows Through Loss.* Grand Rapids: Zondervan Publishing House.
  Sittser lost three generations (daughter, wife, and mother) in a tragic automobile accident. He becomes a single parent who must reconstruct life without three

key females in his life. Circumstances, the author argues, are not important. Rather, it is eternally important what we do with those circumstances!

- Smith, Harold Ivan (1993). *On Grieving the Death of a Father.* Minneapolis: Augsburg. Some 40 persons such as George Bush, Lee Iacocca, Beverly Stills, and Dwight Eisenhower share insights from their experiences of losing a father.

- Smith, Harold Ivan (1996). *Grieving the Death of a Friend.* Minneapolis: Augsburg. Friendgrief is one of the disenfranchised deaths in this culture. More than 10 million people are annually impacted. Over 200 friendgrievers offer insights from their experiences of losing a friend.

- Smith, Harold Ivan (2000). *A Decembered Grief: Living With Loss When Others Are Celebrating.* Kansas City, MO: Beacon Hill Press. Grievers have to survive the triathlon of holidays: Thanksgiving, Christmas, and New Year's. This easy-to-read book offers simple, practical ideas that grievers have found helpful.

- Smith, Harold Ivan (2001). *When Your People Are Grieving: Leading in Times of Loss.* Kansas City, MO: Beacon Hill Press. A comprehensive examination of evangelical Christian pastoral care with particular emphasis on spiritual formation.

- Smith, Harold Ivan (2001). *Friendgrief: An Absence Called Presence.* Amityville, NY: Baywood. An estimated 20 million people each year are directly impacted by the death of a friend. This book examines grief in "the family of investment" and outlines counseling strategies for pastoral care for friendgrievers.

- Smith, Harold Ivan (2004). *Grief Keeping: Learning How Long Grief Lasts.* New York: Crossroad. Death and grief have changed the course of political life at the highest levels in the U.S. In this amazing narrative you will learn the impact of grief processes throughout history in the lives of many U.S. presidents, their families, and other notable American figures.

- Smith, Harold Ivan (2006). *A Long Shadowed Grief: Suicide and its Aftermath.* Boston, MA: Cowley Press. In the aftermath of suicide, family and friends face a long road of grief and reflection. This book ponders the survivor's pains and wondering. He asks how one may live and live out their spirituality.

- Smith, Harold Ivan (2007). *ABC's of Healthy Grieving: Light for a Dark Journey.* Steven L. Jeffers (ed.). Notre Dame, IN: Ave Maria Press. The last thing that a bereaved person is inclined to do is read lengthy, detailed books on how to move though the grief process. *ABC's of Healthy Grieving* is a unique book. It is a document with short, "stand alone," single-page pearls of wisdom on the pilgrimage of grief. It is truly an invaluable and helpful resource.

- Smith, Harold and Johnson, Joy (2006). *What Does That Mean? A Dictionary of Death, Dying and Grief Terms for Grieving Child and Those Who Love Them.* Omaha, NE: The Centering Corporation.

This illustrated dictionary offers child-friendly definitions for more than 150 words associated with death and dying. This book is an important resource for anticipating and answering those tough questions children pose.

- Staudacher, Carol (1991). *Men and Grief: A Guide for Men for Surviving the Death of a Loved One.* Oakland, CA: New Harbinger Publications.
  Contrary to the notion that real men do not grieve, Staudacher counters that they are more likely to work out their grief through activities.

- Staudacher, Carol (1994). *A Time To Grieve: Meditations for Healing After the Death of a Loved One.* San Francisco: Harper.
  Grievers often need to borrow thoughts from others in order to make sense of their own loss. This book offers hundreds of quotations and brief meditations and observations. It is a griever's friend.

- Walter, Tony (1999). *On Bereavement: The Culture of Grief.* Philadelphia: Open University Press.
  This important book examines the social position of the bereaving. Where do they now "fit in" in a society that is aggressively de-ritualizing death?

- Wolfelt, Alan D. (1994). *Creating Meaningful Funeral Rituals: A Guide for Care Givers.* Fort Collins, CO: Compassion Press.
  This book leads funeral service planners and grievers methodically through a most challenging task.

- Yancey, Philip (1990). *Where Is God When It Hurts?* Grand Rapids: Zondervan.
  This classic, originally published in 1977, is an indispensable guide for coping and healing in hard times. Yancey dedicated the most recent printing to those who lost their lives on September 11, 2001, and to their loved ones left behind to wonder why.

Index